Biotech Breakthroughs That Will Change Medicine

By Laura Lee

Inside the Innovations Redefining Health and Human Lifespan

Lauxon Publishing, LLC

Published by Lauxon Publishing, LLC

Introduction:

How Biology Became a Toolkit

Once, medicine's main tools were surprisingly simple: a doctor's hands, a handful of herbs, a knife, a stethoscope, and later, a small pharmacy of chemical drugs. The body was treated as a mostly opaque box. You could listen, press, cut, and prescribe, but there were vast inner regions where cause and effect remained obscure. A fever could be lowered, a pain dulled, a tumor removed, but the underlying instructions that made a body sick or well remained hidden in the tangled code of cells.

Over the last few decades, that code has started to come into view. We have learned to read the letters of DNA, to map which genes turn on in which tissues, and to track how proteins, metabolites, and microbes weave together into the fabric of health. What once seemed like an impenetrable blur is resolving into networks and pathways that we can at least partly understand. The body is still astonishingly complex—and humbling—but it is no longer quite so opaque. Biology has begun to look less like an untouchable mystery and more like a system that, if approached carefully, can be guided and sometimes even reprogrammed.

This book is organized around that shift: from treating symptoms at the surface to working with the underlying systems that generate them. In its early chapters, we explore how medicine is moving from one-size-fits-all approaches to precision and personalization, guided by genomics, big data, and the logic of gene editing. We then move through the living tools of the new era: stem cells that rebuild, immune cells that are trained to hunt disease, microbes that act as partners in metabolism and mood, and organs-on-chips that bring miniature human tissues into the lab. Along the way, we see how synthetic biology, AI, and bioengineering are transforming not only what therapies look like, but how we discover and test them.

The middle of the book turns from inventions to experiences. We look at how biotech shows up at the bedside—in hospitals, infusion centers, and clinics—and how it increasingly flows into homes through wearables, home tests, and direct-to-consumer tools. We explore the promises and pitfalls of editing aging itself, and we pause to consider the ethical questions that arise when life can be engineered: Who decides what counts as "normal." How do we avoid sliding from healing to a quiet form of eugenics. What does fairness mean when some therapies cost more than most people will earn in a lifetime.

The later chapters zoom out even further. They examine access and equity, asking how to prevent a world where some countries and communities enjoy gene therapies and regenerative treatments while others struggle for basic antibiotics and clean water. They look at regulators and safety frameworks, the often-invisible systems that try to ensure that powerful tools are used responsibly. And finally, they follow biotechnology beyond medicine into everyday life—our food, our environment, our jobs—before asking what the next fifty years of medicine might hold if biology continues to become more programmable.

Throughout, this book is written with a simple conviction: understanding the outlines of these technologies should not be reserved for specialists. You do not need to know every molecular detail to grasp the stakes. You only need enough clarity to ask your own questions, to recognize hype when you see it, to understand the options placed in front of you, and to participate in conversations about where we are headed.

Biotech breakthroughs will not just reshape medicine in abstract; they will shape how we are born, how we grow old, how we suffer, and how we heal. They will influence who gets to live longer, who bears which risks, and what kinds of bodies and minds we consider acceptable or desirable. These are not distant, theoretical issues; they are future versions of very intimate decisions. As you move through the chapters ahead, I invite you not only to learn, but also to notice your own reactions—your excitement, your worries, your hopes. The story of biotech is still being written, and your voice is part of how it will unfold.

Table of Contents:

Synthetic Biology and Bioengineering
Scientists are designing new biological systems to solve complex medical problems.

AI as a Lab Partner
Artificial intelligence is accelerating drug discovery, diagnosis, and treatment planning.

Smart Diagnostics and Wearable Health
Wearable devices and smart diagnostics enable continuous monitoring and early detection of disease.

Editing Aging Itself
Longevity science and new therapies aim to extend not just lifespan but also healthspan.

Biotech at the Bedside
Hospitals and clinics are being reshaped by advanced biotech tools and treatments.

At-Home Biotech
Direct-to-consumer tests and digital tools are bringing biotech capabilities into the home.

Ethics in the Age of Engineered Life
Society must decide where to draw the line between treating disease, enhancing humans, and designing life.

Access, Equity, and the Global Biotech Divide
Biotech advances risk widening global inequality unless access gaps are deliberately addressed.

Regulators, Risk, and Responsibility
Laws, policies, and safety frameworks guide, enable, and constrain biotech innovation.

Biotech in Everyday Life
Biotechnology is increasingly shaping our food, environment, and daily experiences beyond traditional medicine.

The Next 50 Years of Medicine

Biology is becoming programmable, opening futures in which medicine is transformed yet again.

Prologue:

Standing at the Edge of the Possible

There are moments in history when the rules of what seems possible quietly change. Most people do not experience these shifts in laboratories or conference halls; they feel them later, in doctor's offices, at kitchen tables, and in the ordinary rituals of caring for one another. The discovery of antibiotics turned once-deadly infections into treatable annoyances. Vaccines moved entire diseases from terrifying inevitabilities to distant memories. Medical imaging gave us the ability to look inside the body without a single incision. Each of these advances began as an improbable idea and ended as something we now take for granted.

We are living through another such moment, though it does not yet have a single name. It is not just about one tool—like CRISPR, or mRNA vaccines, or AI—but about the convergence of many. Genes can be sequenced for less than the price of a plane ticket. Cells can be reprogrammed to grow new tissues or to hunt down cancer. Microbes in our gut are recognized as partners, not just passengers. Algorithms sift through oceans of data, spotting patterns that no human mind could hold alone. Biology, once mysterious and stubbornly analog, is becoming something we can measure, model, and in some cases, deliberately rewrite.

If you listen carefully, you can already hear this shift in the language of medicine. Doctors talk not only about diseases, but about pathways and networks, about the "architecture" of a tumor or the "wiring" of an immune response. They discuss not just side effects, but "off-target" edits, "microbiome signatures," and "digital biomarkers." Patients, too, are changing the conversation, arriving with printouts of genome reports, graphs from wearables, and pointed questions about new therapies they read about online. The old model—where knowledge and power flowed in one direction from expert to patient—is fraying. Something more participatory is emerging in its place.

Yet, for all the headlines and hype, much of what is happening in biotechnology remains hard to see. It sits behind the scenes in the software of hospitals, in the supply chains of drugs, in the quiet routines of labs running thousands of tests a day. It shows up in the timing of a diagnosis, in the precision of a dose, in the decision to watch and wait rather than intervene. The future of medicine does not arrive all at once in a single breakthrough; it seeps into practice one protocol, one device, one decision at a time. Understanding that future means learning to see the hidden scaffolding beneath familiar experiences.

This book is an invitation to step behind the curtain. It will not teach you how to edit a gene or design an organ-on-a-chip. Instead, it will walk you through the landscape of modern biotechnology, showing how its pieces fit together and what they may mean for your health, your community, and the next fifty years of medicine. We will move from the microscopic world of DNA and cells to the macroscopic world of hospitals, homes, and global health systems. Along the way, we will ask questions that are as much about values as about molecules: What counts as a cure. Who gets access. Where do we draw the line between healing and enhancement.

You do not need a scientific background to take this journey. You need only curiosity, a willingness to sit with uncertainty, and an interest in what happens when the boundaries of the possible begin to move. The story of biotech breakthroughs is not just a story about scientists and companies; it is a story about all of us, because it will shape the options available when we or those we love face illness, aging, and the ordinary vulnerabilities of being human. Standing at the edge of the possible, the question is not only what we can do with biology—but who we will become as we do it.

Chapter .1

The Dawn of a New Medical Era

Biotechnology has become the driving engine of modern medicine.

Biotech breakthroughs that will change medicine rarely announce themselves with fanfare in a laboratory. More often, they begin quietly in an exam room, when a doctor opens a chart and sees a kind of information that did not exist for patients a generation ago. Instead of only listing weight, blood pressure, and family history, the record now might include a map of the patient's genes, patterns from a heart monitor worn at home, and predictions generated by software that has studied countless similar cases. For the person sitting on the paper covered table, this is no abstract revolution. It is the moment when medicine stops treating them as an average of everyone and starts seeing them as a singular, complex human being written in molecules and data. That shift, from averages to individuality, is the heartbeat of the biotechnological transformation now sweeping through health care.

Biotechnology, at its core, is the art and science of using living systems to solve human problems. In medicine, those problems include some of the most stubborn challenges our species has ever faced, such as cancer, dementia, and the many chronic illnesses that quietly erode quality of life over decades. For much of the last century, our tools were powerful but blunt, relying on chemicals that affected entire organs or systems in hopes of nudging them toward health. Antibiotics, anesthesia, vaccines, and blood pressure medicines saved countless lives, yet they largely worked without knowing the intimate details of the person receiving them. Today, that is rapidly changing as biologists, engineers, and data scientists learn to read and rewrite the code of life itself. Instead of asking only what disease a patient has, clinicians can increasingly ask what version of a disease this particular body carries and how it might respond to a precisely targeted intervention.

This new medical era did not arrive overnight. It was built through decades of advances in genetics, computing, imaging, and molecular biology, each laying a new layer of understanding on top of the last. When scientists first learned how to copy and sequence fragments of genetic material, it felt like discovering that the body was written in a language, even if no one yet knew how to read all the words. Over time, faster machines, more refined techniques, and vast digital storage turned genetic data from a rare treasure into a common clinical tool. Meanwhile, progress in cell culture, biomaterials, and automation made it possible to grow tissues in dishes and test thousands of potential drugs without ever entering a human bloodstream. These threads have now woven together into a fabric of biotechnology that touches nearly every corner of modern medicine.

To understand why this matters, consider how the traditional model of care treated uncertainty. When a person arrived with a disease, doctors drew on training, experience, and broad statistical studies to pick the treatment most likely to work for most people. If it failed, they would try another approach, and another, adjusting based on how the patient responded over weeks or months. This process could be life saving, but it was also slow, stressful, and sometimes devastating when side effects piled up without delivering real benefit. It was like navigating by a map that only showed the major highways, leaving all the side streets and alleys uncharted. Biotechnology is now filling in those missing details, offering clinicians a more precise map that reflects the unique terrain of each individual.

The new map begins with the genome, the complete set of an individual's genetic instructions. Within that code lie variations that can increase or decrease the risk of disease, alter how a person breaks down a medication, or change how quickly a tumor might grow. Where earlier generations of doctors might have guessed at these hidden factors, today they can often measure them directly. A single test can reveal whether a breast cancer is likely to respond to a particular drug or whether a rare mutation is responsible for a child's unexplained seizures. Instead of treating every case as essentially the same, clinicians can make decisions as if each disease carries a name tag describing its molecular personality. This is the essence of precision medicine, and it is one of the foundations on which the new era rests.

Biotechnology also changes how quickly new treatments can be discovered and improved. In the past, developing a drug often meant many years of trial and error with relatively little feedback from biology until late in the process. Now, researchers can grow miniature versions of organs in the laboratory, test molecules on cells derived from actual patients, and study how diseases progress in living systems that fit on a glass slide. Data from these experiments can be fed into algorithms that search for patterns too complex for any single human mind to notice. Promising compounds can be redesigned at the level of atoms or genes, then tested again, iterating along a tight feedback loop between hypothesis and reality. The result is not just more drugs but smarter, more targeted, and potentially safer therapies.

For patients, these advances often appear first as subtle changes in how care is delivered. A cancer specialist may now send a piece of a tumor to a specialized laboratory before finalizing a treatment plan. A heart doctor might recommend a wearable device that continually tracks rhythms at home, warning of trouble long before symptoms become obvious. A person at high risk for an inherited disorder may undergo genetic counseling and testing to understand their options, including preventive measures that did not exist for their parents. In each case, the underlying technologies are intricate, yet the experience is designed to feel as natural as possible, woven into existing systems rather than replacing them overnight. The transformation is quiet but profound, changing the questions clinicians ask and the answers they can give.

The story of this era is not only written in labs and clinics but also in data centers. Every scan, test, and sensor reading adds a small piece to an enormous mosaic of human health information. When analyzed responsibly and with respect for privacy, this mosaic can reveal trends that were invisible when records were confined to paper folders on dusty shelves. Researchers can compare large groups of cases to see which treatments truly work best for which kinds of people. They can identify early signals of emerging diseases or uncover side effects that only appear in rare combinations of genetics, medications, and environment. In this way, biotechnology and data science together turn the experiences of individual patients into wisdom that can guide care for many others.

Yet even as this progress accelerates, it raises difficult questions. Who will have access to these advanced tests and tailored therapies, and who might be left behind. How do we protect sensitive genetic and health data while still allowing it to be used for the public good. What limits should be placed on editing genes, enhancing traits, or extending human lifespan beyond anything seen before. These questions reach far beyond the boundaries of medicine, touching on ethics, law, economics, and cultural values. Any honest account of the new medical era must acknowledge that it offers both extraordinary hope and serious responsibility.

The chapters that follow trace the major strands of this transformation. They explore how precision therapies work, how gene editing tools are entering the clinic, how stem cells and regenerative strategies aim to repair the body from within, and how the immune system can be taught to fight cancer more effectively. They examine the hidden worlds of the microbiome and living models grown on chips, and they describe how artificial intelligence assists scientists at the bench and clinicians at the bedside. They also grapple with the dilemmas of access, regulation, and equity, because no breakthrough is truly complete if it cannot reach those who need it most. Each topic could fill its own volume, yet here they are woven into a single story about where medicine is heading and what it may feel like to live in that future. As you read, you are invited not just to learn about these tools but to imagine how they might reshape your own experience of health, illness, and care.

Author Reflection

When I think about the dawn of this new medical era, I am struck by how ordinary it can look from the outside. A blood draw, a smartwatch notification, or a line in a medical chart can mask the decades of labor, curiosity, and persistence that made it possible. Writing this chapter reminded me that breakthroughs are rarely sudden miracles, but the cumulative result of many people asking better questions about the same old problems. At the same time, I feel a deep humility, because every new tool can be used wisely or carelessly, generously or selfishly. My hope is that by pulling back the curtain on these technologies, this book helps readers feel less intimidated by science and more empowered to join conversations about how it should be used. The future of medicine is not only in the hands of experts in white coats; it is also in the values and choices of all of us who will one day be patients, caregivers, and citizens shaping the rules.

Inspirational Quotes

Every medical breakthrough begins as a question no one was entirely sure it was worth asking.

Chapter .2

From Pills to Precision

Healthcare is shifting from one-size-fits-all treatments to highly tailored, personalized therapies.

For most of modern history, medicine has relied on a simple question: what generally works for most people with this condition. When someone had high blood pressure, a doctor chose from a short list of drugs shown to help large groups of patients in clinical trials. If the first pill did not work or caused side effects, they tried another, and then another, slowly feeling their way toward something that fit. This approach saved lives and extended lifespans across the world, but it carried an invisible cost in trial and error. Many patients endured months or years of suboptimal care before reaching the right combination of treatments. Beneath the surface of those averages, biology was quietly reminding us that no two bodies are truly the same.

Precision medicine arises from the realization that those differences are not a nuisance to be ignored, but a map to be read. Instead of assuming that everyone with the same diagnosis should get the same treatment, precision medicine asks what makes this particular person's disease unique. That uniqueness might lie in their genes, the way their liver processes drugs, the composition of their microbiome, or the environment in which they live and work.

Each factor can influence whether a therapy helps, harms, or does nothing at all. By measuring these influences and building them into decisions, clinicians can move from guessing to guiding. The goal is not perfection, but a steady narrowing of uncertainty so that fewer patients must suffer through long stretches of trial and error.

One of the clearest examples of this shift is in oncology, the treatment of cancer. In the past, cancers were mainly classified by where they appeared in the body and how they looked under a microscope. A lung tumor and a breast tumor were considered fundamentally different, and patients were offered standard combinations of surgery, radiation, and chemotherapy. Today, those visual clues are only the beginning of the story. Tumors are often analyzed at the molecular level to identify mutations, signaling pathways, and surface markers that drive their growth. Two cancers from different organs might share the same mutation and respond to the same targeted drug, while two lung cancers might differ so much at the molecular level that they need completely different strategies. Precision oncology does not replace traditional tools, but it layers new information on top of them to sharpen the aim.

Pharmacogenomics, the study of how genes affect a person's response to medications, is another key pillar of this new approach. Many people know someone who has tried an antidepressant that did nothing, or a pain medication that made them nauseated without touching their discomfort. These experiences once felt mysterious, as if some people simply had "bad luck" with certain drugs. Now we know that variations in genes coding for enzymes, transporters, and receptors can dramatically shape how a medicine behaves in the body. Some people break down a drug so quickly that it never reaches a therapeutic level, while others process it so slowly that even a normal dose becomes toxic. By testing for specific genetic variants, clinicians can sometimes choose better starting doses or avoid certain drugs entirely for those at high risk of side effects.

Beyond genetics, precision medicine also draws on rich streams of data from imaging, laboratory tests, and digital monitoring. An individual with heart failure, for instance, can be monitored through implanted sensors or wearable devices that capture heart rhythms, fluid levels, and activity patterns over time. These data can reveal early warning signs of deterioration long before the person feels short of breath. Algorithms can flag these changes and prompt clinicians to adjust medications or recommend a visit, preventing hospitalizations that once seemed inevitable. The precision here lies not in a single magic test, but in combining many small signals into a clear picture of how a particular heart is coping with daily life.

Electronic health records, for all their frustrations, also play an important role in enabling more personalized care. They offer a centralized place where genetics, imaging, labs, medications, and clinical notes can be linked and analyzed together. When designed and used thoughtfully, they allow patterns to emerge across large populations while still highlighting what makes an individual unique. For example, a system might compare a patient's lab results and treatment history to thousands of others with similar profiles, suggesting therapies that led to better outcomes in that specific group. This does not replace the judgment of clinicians, but it gives them additional lenses through which to interpret complex cases. It is as if the accumulated experience of many doctors and patients could be consulted at once, distilled into guidance for the person in front of you.

Precision medicine is not only about high-tech tools; it also changes the questions clinicians ask during everyday encounters. Rather than focusing solely on the disease, they may spend more time understanding lifestyle, family history, and personal goals. A treatment that is optimal on paper may not fit a person's values, schedule, or tolerance for risk. A young parent might accept a more aggressive therapy with harsher side effects if it offers a better chance of long-term survival, while an older patient might prioritize comfort and independence over an extra few months of life. Precision care acknowledges that the "right" treatment must be biologically appropriate and personally meaningful. In this sense, personalization is as much about listening as it is about measuring.

The rise of personalized therapies also changes how we think about prevention. In the past, public health advice tended to be broad and universal: eat more vegetables, exercise regularly, avoid smoking, and get screened at certain ages. These recommendations remain important and evidence based, yet they do not capture the full range of risk that individuals face. Someone with a strong genetic predisposition to a given cancer might need earlier and more frequent screening than standard guidelines suggest. Another person's genes might protect them in one area but make them more vulnerable to heart disease or diabetes. By integrating genetic risk scores, family history, and environmental exposures, clinicians can design prevention plans that target the specific threats most likely to matter for each person.

However, precision medicine is not a magic solution that instantly eliminates all uncertainty. Many genetic variants have subtle or poorly understood effects, and not every test result leads to a clear clinical action. Sometimes, screening uncovers mutations associated with moderately increased risk, leaving patients and clinicians to wrestle with probabilities rather than clear yes or no answers. Overdiagnosis and overtreatment can become real concerns if uncertain findings lead to aggressive interventions that may not be necessary. Precision care therefore requires humility, clear communication, and shared decision making. It asks clinicians to explain what is known, what is not, and how comfortable they are with different options, then invites patients into the conversation as partners.

The economics of precision medicine also present a complex picture. Some of the most advanced tests and therapies are expensive, and they often emerge first in wealthy health systems and academic centers. Targeted cancer drugs and gene-based diagnostics can strain budgets and raise difficult questions about what societies are willing or able to pay. At the same time, more precise care has the potential to reduce waste by avoiding treatments unlikely to work and preventing costly complications. A single hospitalization avoided, a surgery rendered unnecessary, or a drug reaction prevented can offset significant costs. As technologies mature, prices often fall, making them accessible to broader populations. The challenge lies in managing the transition, ensuring that innovation does not deepen existing disparities in health.

Ethical considerations are woven throughout the shift from pills to precision. When genetic information becomes part of routine care, concerns about privacy, discrimination, and consent move to the forefront. People may worry that their data could be used by insurers, employers, or others in ways that harm them. They may wonder whether they truly want to know their risk for certain diseases, especially when preventive options are limited. In response, many countries have developed laws and guidelines to safeguard genetic data and limit its misuse, but the technology often evolves faster than policy. Maintaining trust requires not only regulations but also transparent communication about who can access data, for what purposes, and how it will be protected.

Another ethical question arises around the concept of "normal." As we get better at measuring individual differences, we may be tempted to label more variations as problems to be fixed. A genetic variant that slightly raises risk for a condition might be framed as a defect rather than a natural part of human diversity. Precision tools can sharpen this temptation, offering the illusion that every deviation from average health is an error in need of correction. Resisting this mindset requires remembering that variation is the raw material of evolution and individuality. Medicine's purpose is not to turn everyone into the same idealized model, but to support people in living full, meaningful lives in bodies that will always be imperfect.

Education and communication are crucial if precision medicine is to fulfill its promise. Complex concepts like gene expression, risk scores, and targeted therapies must be translated into language that patients and families can understand and use. This does not mean oversimplifying or hiding uncertainty; it means building bridges between technical knowledge and everyday experience. Clinicians might use analogies, visual aids, or decision tools that let patients explore "what if" scenarios. Patients, in turn, can learn to ask new kinds of questions: how was this recommendation generated, what data support it, and how does it align with my own goals and concerns. In this way, precision is not something done to patients but something built with them.

Finally, the shift from pills to precision changes how we imagine the future of medicine itself. Instead of picturing a world where every disease has a single definitive cure, we might envision a landscape of many small, tailored solutions that evolve over time. Treatments may be adjusted dynamically as new data arrive, much like navigation apps recalculating a route when traffic conditions change. Some diseases may be prevented or softened rather than eliminated outright. The measure of success will be not only how long people live but how long they can pursue their passions, maintain relationships, and participate in their communities. Precision medicine, at its best, is not a cold exercise in categorization but a warmer, more attentive way of caring for human beings in all their complexity.

If the first era of modern medicine was defined by powerful but generalized pills, the emerging era is defined by the integration of detailed knowledge about individuals into every stage of care. The journey from pills to precision is still unfolding, with uneven access, unanswered questions, and many technical challenges ahead. Nevertheless, its direction is clear. We are moving away from treating patients as interchangeable and toward honoring the specific biology and biography each person brings into the clinic. As we do, medicine becomes less a game of odds and more a practice of understanding. In the chapters ahead, we will look more closely at the tools that make this possible, beginning with the ability to decode the human blueprint written in our DNA.

Chapter .3

Decoding the Human Blueprint

Genomics and big data are revealing what our DNA can tell us about health and disease.

The idea that the body carries a blueprint has fascinated scientists and philosophers for centuries. For most of history, that blueprint was a metaphor, invoked to describe the mysterious instructions that turned a single cell into a complex human being. Today, it is a literal description of the sequences of DNA that reside in almost every cell of our bodies. Those sequences, written in four chemical letters, encode the recipes for proteins, the regulators that control their production, and many other elements that shape our development and function. When people talk about the human genome, they are referring to the full set of these instructions, taken together as a single, immense text. Decoding that text has become one of the central projects of modern biology and a cornerstone of the new medicine.

The completion of the first human genome sequence at the beginning of this century was a turning point in this story. It required the work of thousands of researchers, massive investments, and machines that were state of the art for their time. The effort took many years and cost billions of dollars, which made it a feat that only nations and large organizations could attempt. Yet the result was more than a single reference genome; it was proof that such a map could be made at all. Once the first map existed, scientists could begin to compare it with the genomes of many other individuals to see how people differ at the level of DNA. Those differences, scattered like spelling variations across billions of letters, hold clues to why some people get sick while others remain healthy.

Technological innovation quickly began to shrink the cost and time required to sequence DNA. New methods emerged that could read millions of short fragments in parallel and then use computational tools to assemble them into a coherent sequence. As machines improved and competition increased, what once took years could be done in days, and what once cost fortunes became roughly comparable to the price of a major medical test. This shift turned genome sequencing from a rare research endeavor into something that could plausibly be used in clinical care. It also meant that researchers could undertake projects that compared the genomes of tens or hundreds of thousands of people. The scale of available data grew from a trickle to a flood, calling for new ways to organize, analyze, and interpret it.

At its simplest, a genome sequence is a long list of the positions of the four DNA bases in an individual. On its own, that list is not very informative, because no mind can grasp the meaning of billions of letters by simple inspection. The power of genomics comes from comparing many such lists to each other and to a reference, looking for systematic differences that correlate with traits or diseases. These differences, often single base changes known as variants, can be harmless, harmful, or beneficial, depending on where they occur and what they alter. Some variants disrupt the function of crucial genes and lead to rare, severe conditions. Others subtly tweak the regulation of genes, nudging the risk of common diseases a little higher or lower. Sorting out which variants matter and in what ways is one of the central challenges of modern genomics.

Large population studies have become a key tool in addressing that challenge. In such studies, scientists collect genetic data from many individuals along with information about their health, lifestyle, and environment. They then use statistical methods to identify associations between specific variants and specific traits, such as blood pressure, cholesterol levels, or the presence of disease. These analyses can reveal that people carrying a particular variant are more likely than others to develop a certain condition. They can also show that some genetic influences are shared across multiple diseases, hinting at common underlying pathways. While association does not prove causation, it often points to biological mechanisms worth deeper investigation.

One of the surprising lessons from these studies is that many common diseases are influenced by a very large number of genetic variants, each contributing a small effect. Instead of a single mutation that determines destiny, people often carry many variants that together shape their risk in complex ways. To make sense of this, researchers have developed methods to calculate combined measures known as polygenic risk scores. These scores sum the weight of thousands of small genetic influences into a single number that reflects relative risk compared to the general population. Such scores are not perfect predictions, and they must be interpreted carefully in context. Still, they offer a glimpse into how the blueprint of DNA can help identify people who may benefit from more intensive screening or early preventive measures.

Genomics has been particularly transformative in the realm of rare diseases. For families who have spent years seeking answers for unexplained symptoms, a genome or exome sequence can sometimes provide a long-awaited diagnosis. By scanning the coding regions of genes for disruptive variants, clinicians can uncover previously hidden causes of developmental disorders, metabolic conditions, or neurological problems. In some cases, the discovery leads to specific treatments or dietary changes that dramatically improve quality of life. In others, it does not change therapy but gives families clarity about what they are facing and how it might affect future children. Even when the findings do not fully resolve a mystery, they add to a growing body of knowledge that may benefit others in the future.

Another important application of decoding the human blueprint lies in carrier screening and reproductive decision making. Couples who are planning to have children can undergo testing to see whether they both carry harmful variants in the same gene. If they do, their offspring may be at significant risk for a recessive genetic disease. Knowing this in advance allows them to explore options such as in vitro fertilization with genetic testing of embryos or the use of donor gametes. These choices are deeply personal and can be emotionally complex. Genomic information does not dictate what couples should do, but it gives them more information with which to weigh their values, hopes, and fears.

Genomics also intersects with wellness and identity in ways that go beyond strict medical care. Direct to consumer genetic tests have become widely available, offering people insights into ancestry, certain traits, and limited health related information. Many people are curious about where their ancestors came from and how their genetic heritage compares to others around the world. Others are interested in learning about genetic variants linked to traits such as lactose tolerance or taste perception. While these offerings can be engaging and sometimes enlightening, they also come with limitations and risks of misunderstanding. Not all reported associations are equally strong, and the significance of some findings can be exaggerated in marketing materials.

Understanding what genomic results actually mean requires careful interpretation. A report that someone carries a variant associated with moderately increased risk for a disease does not mean that they will definitely develop it. Environmental factors, lifestyle choices, and chance all continue to play large roles in health outcomes. Conversely, a lack of known high risk variants does not guarantee safety from illness. The genome is a map of possibilities, not a fixed script. Communicating this nuance is essential to help people avoid fatalism or false reassurance. Clinicians and genetic counselors can act as guides, helping individuals integrate genomic information with other aspects of their lives and health.

The rise of genomics has also transformed research into how medicines work. By examining which variants are more common in people who respond well or poorly to a particular drug, scientists can identify genetic factors that influence drug metabolism or sensitivity. This field, closely related to pharmacogenomics, helps explain why a standard dose can be too much for one person and not enough for another. It also guides the design of new drugs that target specific pathways implicated by genetic studies. In this way, decoding the blueprint does not only reveal why diseases occur; it also points toward new strategies for intervention. The genome thus becomes a roadmap for drug discovery as well as diagnosis.

Big data and genomics are deeply intertwined. Modern sequencing projects generate massive amounts of information, often measured in terabytes or more, which must be stored, curated, and analyzed. To handle this volume, researchers rely on sophisticated computational infrastructure and algorithms. Machine learning techniques can sift through complex patterns of variation and help distinguish signal from noise. Cloud computing enables collaborations across institutions and countries, allowing diverse datasets to be combined in ways that increase their power. These technological advances make it possible to ask questions that would have been unthinkable when genomes were first being mapped.

One important development has been the creation of large biobanks and cohort studies that link genomic data with detailed health records. Participants in these initiatives consent to having their DNA analyzed and their clinical information used for research, often over many years. As their health journeys unfold, new diagnoses, treatments, and outcomes are added to the database. Researchers can then examine how genetic factors interact with medications, surgeries, or lifestyle changes over time. This dynamic view reveals not only who is at risk for certain diseases but also how different interventions alter the course of illness. It advances our understanding of the blueprint as something that is constantly interpreted by the body in changing environments.

Despite these achievements, significant gaps remain in our genomic knowledge. Many early studies focused disproportionately on populations of European ancestry, leaving people from other backgrounds underrepresented in the data. This imbalance can lead to risk models and interpretations that work less well for large portions of the world's population. It also means that potentially important variants specific to certain groups may go unnoticed. Addressing these gaps requires deliberate efforts to include diverse participants and to build trust with communities historically excluded or harmed by research. When done well, such inclusion not only advances science but also promotes fairness in the benefits that genomic medicine can provide.

There are also many parts of the genome whose functions are still poorly understood. While protein coding genes have been studied intensively, large stretches of non coding DNA play regulatory roles that are only beginning to be mapped. These regions act like switches, dimmers, and timers that control when and where genes are turned on or off. Variants in regulatory elements can influence disease risk by altering the levels of key proteins rather than changing their structure. Understanding this regulatory landscape requires integrating genomic data with measurements of RNA, proteins, and chromatin structure in different cell types. The blueprint, in other words, is not just a list of parts but a dynamic script that changes over time and context.

Epigenetics adds another layer of complexity to this picture. Epigenetic marks are chemical changes to DNA and its associated proteins that affect how genes are expressed without altering the underlying sequence. They can be influenced by development, environment, stress, and behavior. Unlike sequence variants, some epigenetic changes are reversible, and a few can even be passed down across generations. Studying these patterns helps explain how experiences such as malnutrition or toxin exposure can leave biological traces that shape long term health. It also offers new avenues for therapy by targeting the enzymes that place or remove these marks. When we talk about decoding the human blueprint, we are increasingly including these epigenetic annotations alongside the genetic text.

Privacy and security are central concerns in the age of genomic big data. A genome is deeply personal information, and it can reveal details not only about the individual but also about their relatives. Even when data are stripped of obvious identifiers, patterns in the sequences can sometimes be used to re identify people under certain conditions. Safeguarding genomic databases therefore requires strong technical protections, strict policies, and clear ethical guidelines. It also requires ongoing dialogue with participants about the risks and benefits of contributing their data. Trust is fragile, and once broken it can be difficult to repair, so transparency about how genomic information is used is essential.

Law and policy are evolving to keep pace with genomic advances. Many regions have enacted regulations to limit genetic discrimination in employment and insurance, seeking to ensure that people are not penalized for information they did not choose. Research ethics frameworks have been updated to address questions about returning results to participants and handling incidental findings. Courts have weighed in on issues such as the patenting of genes and the ownership of biological samples. These legal developments shape the environment in which scientists and clinicians operate. They also influence how comfortable people feel about engaging with genomic technologies in their own lives.

Cultural perspectives play a significant role in how societies respond to the promise and challenges of genomics. In some communities, genetic explanations for disease may resonate with existing beliefs about ancestry, fate, or family. In others, they may clash with spiritual or philosophical views of health and identity. Different cultures have varied experiences with medical research, including histories of exploitation or neglect, that color their trust in new technologies. Decoding the human blueprint is therefore not simply a scientific or technical project. It is also a social and cultural conversation about what it means to know so much about our biological selves.

Education is crucial if individuals and communities are to navigate this new landscape. Schools, media, and public health organizations all have roles to play in explaining basic genomic concepts in accessible ways. People do not need to become experts in molecular biology to make informed decisions, but they do need foundational understanding of what genes are and how risk works. Clinicians can support this learning by building genomic literacy into routine care and by collaborating with genetic counselors. As knowledge spreads, the public becomes better equipped to participate in policy debates, research governance, and personal health choices related to genomics.

Decoding the human blueprint also reshapes how we think about the boundaries between health and disease. Some genetic variants confer high risk for specific conditions, but most are neither purely good nor purely bad in every context. A variant that increases susceptibility to one disease might protect against another. Traits once considered purely environmental may turn out to have genetic components, while others thought to be inheritable may be more influenced by social factors. These insights challenge simple narratives and call for a more nuanced understanding of causation. They remind us that biology is intertwined with environment and society at every level.

The expanding ability to read genomes raises the question of whether we should also rewrite them, a topic explored in more detail in later chapters. For now, it is enough to note that understanding the blueprint is a prerequisite for any attempt to edit it safely. The more precisely we can map the consequences of variants, the better we can anticipate the effects of proposed changes. This does not mean that every edit will be predictable, but it does create a foundation for responsible experimentation. In this sense, genomics is both an end in itself and a stepping stone toward more active interventions in the machinery of life.

Ultimately, decoding the human blueprint is about more than diagnosing disease or developing new therapies. It offers a deeper appreciation of the shared heritage that connects all people, as well as the variations that make each individual unique. It invites us to see ourselves as part of a continuous story written across generations, with each genome carrying echoes of ancestors and whispers of potential futures. At the same time, it underscores the limits of biological determinism by highlighting the importance of environment, chance, and choice. The genome is a powerful influence, but it is not destiny. How we live, what we build, and how we care for one another continue to shape health in profound ways.

As genomics and big data continue to mature, their integration into everyday medicine will deepen. Newborns may routinely receive genomic screening to identify conditions that can be treated early, while adults may have their genomes referenced throughout their lives as new discoveries emerge. Treatments may be guided by risk algorithms that blend genetic, clinical, and environmental data into personalized forecasts. Researchers will continue to unveil connections between genes and traits that were once invisible. All of this will require ongoing attention to equity, ethics, and communication. It will also require a willingness to revisit assumptions as new evidence accumulates.

In the broader arc of this book, the decoding of the human blueprint provides the foundation on which many other breakthroughs rest. Gene editing tools, gene therapies, and targeted drugs all rely on detailed knowledge of how genes function and interact. Understanding the microbiome, the immune system, and aging itself is enriched by genomic insights. Even technologies that operate outside the body, such as organs on chips and artificial intelligence systems for drug discovery, draw heavily on genomic data. By mapping the instructions of life, we have opened a new chapter in the story of medicine. The next chapters will show how we are beginning to write back into that story, altering genes, cells, and systems in the hope of healing and, in some cases, transforming what it means to be ill.

Chapter .4

CRISPR and the Gene-Editing Revolution

CRISPR technology is being used to rewrite faulty genes to prevent and cure disease.

When people first hear the phrase "gene editing," it can sound like science fiction, as if someone has discovered an editorial pen for the code of life. At a basic level, that image is not far from the truth. Every cell in the body carries long strands of DNA, where genes are written in sequences of four chemical letters. For most of human history, those letters were fixed, passed down from parent to child with only rare, random changes. Medicine could respond to the consequences of harmful mutations but had no way to reach back into the DNA itself and correct them. CRISPR changed that by offering a comparatively simple, precise way to cut and modify genes directly inside living cells.

CRISPR's story begins not in human laboratories but in bacteria. For years, microbiologists studying bacterial DNA noticed odd repeating patterns separated by unique sequences, like a chorus with different verses between each refrain. These strange regions turned out to be part of a bacterial immune system that remembers viruses and defends against them. When a virus attacks, the bacterium can capture a small piece of its DNA and store it between the repeats as a genetic mugshot. Later, if the same virus appears again, the bacterium uses that stored sequence, along with special proteins, to recognize and slice the invader's DNA. This natural defense mechanism is what we now call CRISPR, an acronym for "clustered regularly interspaced short palindromic repeats."

The key insight that sparked the gene-editing revolution was that this microbial system could be repurposed as a programmable tool. Scientists realized they could design a small piece of RNA to guide the CRISPR machinery to almost any desired DNA sequence. The Cas9 protein, often described as molecular scissors, would then make a cut at that precise location in the genome. Once the DNA is cut, the cell's own repair systems rush in to fix the break. By influencing how that repair happens, researchers can disrupt a gene, insert a new sequence, or correct a faulty one. Suddenly, editing genes in many types of cells became more accessible, more flexible, and cheaper than with earlier techniques.

Before CRISPR, gene editing was possible but cumbersome and technically demanding. Methods like zinc finger nucleases and TALENs required custom-designed proteins for each target, which made every new project laborious and expensive. CRISPR, by contrast, separated the cutting machinery from the targeting instructions. The Cas9 protein could stay the same while only the guide RNA had to be changed to aim at a new location. It was like moving from chiseling words into stone to typing them into a computer: the basic act remained similar, but the speed and versatility increased dramatically. This shift opened the door to thousands of laboratories around the world, not just a specialized few, and unleashed a wave of experimentation.

The simplest use of CRISPR in the lab is to "knock out" a gene, meaning to disable it so scientists can observe what happens. By introducing a cut and letting the cell repair it in a sloppy way, small errors are introduced that often break the gene's function. If the cell's behavior changes in a particular way after the knockout, researchers gain clues about what that gene normally does. By systematically knocking out genes one by one across the genome, it becomes possible to map networks of interactions that underlie processes like cell division, metabolism, and immune responses. In this sense, CRISPR is not only a therapeutic tool but also a powerful engine for basic discovery.

Turning CRISPR from a research instrument into a medical therapy requires an extra layer of complexity. It is one thing to edit cells growing in a dish, and quite another to reach targeted cells deep inside a human body. For many potential treatments, scientists must find safe ways to deliver CRISPR components to specific tissues, such as bone marrow, liver, or the retina. They also need to control when and how long the machinery is active, so it makes the desired changes but does not linger where it is no longer needed. Different strategies exist, including packaging CRISPR in viral vectors, sending it in as RNA or protein complexes, or editing cells outside the body and then returning them to the patient. Each approach has trade-offs in safety, efficiency, and practicality.

Some of the earliest and most promising CRISPR therapies focus on diseases caused by relatively simple genetic errors. Sickle cell disease, for example, results from a single-letter change in the gene that encodes part of hemoglobin, the protein that carries oxygen in red blood cells. This tiny alteration causes hemoglobin to clump under low-oxygen conditions, deforming red cells into rigid sickle shapes that block blood vessels and damage tissues. Patients endure episodes of intense pain, increased risk of infection, and shortened lifespans. CRISPR-based treatments aim either to correct the faulty gene directly or to reactivate a fetal form of hemoglobin that can compensate for the defect. Early clinical results have shown that some patients who received edited cells experienced dramatic reductions in painful crises.

Inherited blindness offers another example of CRISPR's therapeutic potential. Certain forms of vision loss are caused by mutations in specific genes that affect cells in the retina, the light-sensitive tissue at the back of the eye. Because the eye is relatively accessible and somewhat immune-privileged, it has long been considered a good candidate for gene therapy. CRISPR adds the ability to make precise edits inside retinal cells, potentially restoring or preserving function in ways that traditional treatments cannot. While not every case of blindness can be addressed this way, these efforts illustrate how gene editing can be tailored to the unique biology of particular tissues. They also show how even partial improvements in function can have life-changing impact for patients.

CRISPR is not limited to fixing malfunctioning genes; it can also be used to enhance the way cells fight disease. In cancer therapy, for instance, researchers have explored using CRISPR to engineer immune cells so they recognize and attack tumors more effectively. One strategy involves collecting a patient's T cells, editing them to better identify cancer cells or resist suppression, and then infusing them back into the bloodstream. Another strategy edits immune cells from donors to create off-the-shelf therapies that can be used for many patients, with modifications to reduce the risk of rejection. These approaches build on earlier forms of cellular immunotherapy but add CRISPR's precision to refine the cells' behavior.

Despite its power, CRISPR is not a perfect tool, and its limitations matter greatly in the context of medicine. One concern is the possibility of off-target effects, where the editing machinery cuts DNA at unintended sites that resemble the intended target. Even rare unintended changes could potentially disrupt important genes or trigger harmful effects in the long term. To address this, scientists have developed improved versions of Cas proteins with higher specificity and have refined guide RNA design to reduce mismatches. They also use extensive sequencing to check for unexpected edits in cells before using them therapeutically. The goal is to minimize risk without giving up the transformative benefits that precise editing can offer.

Another challenge lies in controlling exactly what happens after CRISPR makes a cut. Cells can repair breaks in DNA using several different pathways, some of which are more predictable than others. For simple gene knockouts, the error-prone repair process is actually helpful, since small disruptive changes are sufficient. For precise corrections, however, researchers often want the cell to use a template that provides the correct sequence to copy in. Encouraging cells to choose this high-fidelity pathway has proven difficult, especially in non-dividing cells. New gene-editing technologies, such as base editors and prime editors, have been developed to address this, allowing changes to be made without cutting both strands of the DNA. These innovations extend the CRISPR concept and illustrate how rapidly the field continues to evolve.

Ethics loom large whenever people discuss gene editing, especially when the possibility of altering future generations enters the conversation. Somatic editing, which targets cells in an individual's body without affecting eggs or sperm, impacts only that person and is generally seen as more acceptable when aimed at treating serious disease. Germline editing, by contrast, would change the genome in ways that can be inherited by descendants. Many scientists and ethicists argue that germline interventions should not be attempted at this time, given the scientific uncertainties and profound societal implications. International bodies and national academies have called for broad public dialogue and strong regulation to prevent premature or unethical use. The controversy surrounding early, unauthorized germline experiments has only sharpened these concerns.

Decisions about how and when to use CRISPR touch deeply on questions of fairness and access. If powerful gene-editing treatments are developed, there is a risk they will be available first to those who are already privileged. That could create a world in which genetic advantages layer on top of existing social and economic inequalities. Even within healthcare systems, choices about which diseases to target and which populations to prioritize will reflect values and biases. Some worry about a drift toward "enhancement" applications, where traits such as height, cognition, or appearance are altered to fit narrow ideals. Drawing clear lines between therapy and enhancement is not always simple, but many agree that preventing suffering from serious disease should remain the primary focus, at least in the near term.

Public understanding and engagement are essential for navigating these ethical landscapes. CRISPR is a highly technical tool, yet its consequences will affect entire societies, not just experts. People need accessible explanations of what gene editing can and cannot do, what risks it carries, and what safeguards are in place. They also deserve a voice in setting the rules that guide research and clinical use. Toward this end, forums, citizen assemblies, and cross-cultural dialogues have begun to emerge, inviting individuals from diverse backgrounds to explore their hopes and fears about genetic technologies. These conversations will likely continue for decades as new capabilities arise.

CRISPR's influence extends beyond human medicine into agriculture, ecology, and basic biology, blurring the boundaries of what counts as "medical" biotechnology. Crops may be edited for resilience to climate change, pests, or nutrient deficiencies, potentially improving food security. Disease-carrying insects could be targeted with gene drives that bias inheritance to reduce their populations or render them harmless, though such interventions carry ecological risks. Microbes can be engineered to produce pharmaceuticals, biofuels, or materials more efficiently. In each case, the underlying logic is similar: use CRISPR to make targeted changes that unlock new functions or suppress harmful ones. These applications remind us that gene editing is a general-purpose tool whose societal impact will be broad.

For individual patients, however, the meaning of CRISPR is often intensely personal. It may be the difference between a life hemmed in by repeated hospitalizations and one with far fewer medical crises. It can represent an answer to a long-standing "why" behind a family's health struggles and a glimpse of a different future for the next generation. At the same time, not every disease will be easily addressed by editing a single gene, and not every person will want or be able to access such treatments. Managing expectations is therefore critical. CRISPR is a powerful addition to the medical toolbox, but it is not a panacea that will instantly cure all genetic illness.

Looking ahead, the gene-editing revolution is likely to unfold in stages. Early therapies will probably remain focused on conditions where the biology is relatively straightforward, the affected cells are accessible, and the benefits clearly outweigh the risks. As techniques improve, more complex diseases and tissues may come within reach. Along the way, regulators, clinicians, and communities will need to revisit guidelines as evidence accumulates. New editing platforms may supplant or augment current CRISPR systems, just as CRISPR itself supplanted older tools. The revolution, in other words, is not a single event but an ongoing process of refinement and learning.

In the wider story of this book, CRISPR sits at the hinge between reading the human blueprint and rewriting it. Genomics gives us the language and the grammar, revealing which changes are linked to which traits and diseases. Gene editing supplies the ability to correct, adjust, or explore that code in living cells. Together, they transform medicine from a discipline that mainly responds to biology into one that can increasingly reprogram it. The next chapter turns from tools that change genes to therapies that deliver those changes into people's lives, showing how gene editing and related technologies are already moving from the lab bench into real-world clinical practice.

Chapter .5

Gene Therapies in Action

Real-world stories show how conditions once considered untreatable are being transformed by gene therapy.

There is a particular kind of silence that fills a room when a doctor says, "We have something new to try." For many families living with rare genetic diseases, that sentence once seemed impossible, because there was nothing new to offer beyond supportive care and hope. Gene therapy has begun to change that by targeting illnesses at their molecular roots, rather than only managing symptoms on the surface. Instead of asking how to help the body cope with a missing or broken protein, clinicians can now ask whether it is possible to provide the correct genetic instructions so that protein can be made again. This shift turns the story of treatment from an endless cycle of daily medications into the possibility of a single, transformative intervention. The cases where this has already happened are not fairy tales; they are medical records, lived experiences, and the foundations of a rapidly growing field.

To understand gene therapy in practice, it helps to see how it differs from traditional drugs. Conventional medications are usually small molecules or biological products that act on proteins or pathways already present in the body. Their effects last only as long as the drug remains at effective levels, which is why many conditions require lifelong treatment. Gene therapy, by contrast, aims to insert, repair, or regulate the genetic instructions themselves inside cells. Once those instructions are in place, the cell can, in principle, make the needed protein for months or years without further intervention. This does not guarantee a permanent cure, but it opens the door to long-lasting benefits after a single dose. For many patients, that difference feels like the contrast between renting health and owning a piece of it.

One of the most striking demonstrations of gene therapy's power has come in treating spinal muscular atrophy, a devastating disease that affects motor neurons. Babies born with severe forms of this condition gradually lose the ability to move, swallow, and ultimately breathe, because the nerve cells that control muscles degenerate. For years, the prognosis was heartbreaking, with many children dying in early infancy despite all available care. Gene therapy approaches target the missing or malfunctioning gene responsible for producing a crucial survival motor neuron protein. By delivering a functional copy of this gene to motor neurons, clinicians can change the trajectory of the disease in a way that once seemed unimaginable. Parents who expected to plan for hospice now find themselves watching their children reach milestones like sitting, standing, or even walking.

These improvements do not erase every limitation or risk. Gene therapy for spinal muscular atrophy is complex to administer, closely monitored, and not without side effects. The immune system may react to the viral vectors that carry the new genetic material, and liver function must be watched carefully. Some children respond more robustly than others, depending on how early treatment is started and how much damage has already occurred. Yet even with these caveats, the contrast between treated and untreated cases is stark. What was once an almost uniformly fatal diagnosis now has a growing record of children living longer and more active lives. In clinical photos and videos, one can see the practical meaning of molecular medicine in bright eyes, curious hands, and wobbly first steps.

Inherited retinal diseases provide another window into gene therapy in action. Certain forms of blindness arise when a specific gene in the retinal cells is defective, leaving the light-sensitive tissue unable to process visual signals correctly. People with these conditions often experience night blindness, narrowing fields of vision, and progressive loss of sight, sometimes starting in childhood. For one such condition, a gene therapy was developed that delivers a correct copy of the faulty gene directly to retinal cells through a carefully controlled injection. After treatment, some patients have reported being able to navigate in low light for the first time, recognize faces more easily, or see colors that had faded into a dim blur. Clinical tests confirm measurable improvements in visual function, even if vision is not restored to perfection.

The emotional impact of these changes is hard to capture in statistics alone. Imagine a teenager who has grown accustomed to clinging to railings in the dark suddenly walking more confidently at dusk. Picture a child who once avoided dimly lit rooms now insisting on turning off the lights to show how well they can see. For families, these moments are not just clinical milestones; they are deeply human experiences that reshape daily life. They also underscore a crucial point about gene therapy's goals. In many cases, the aim is not to produce flawless, textbook-normal function, but to restore enough capacity to make meaningful differences in independence, safety, and joy. A few lines of corrected genetic code can ripple outward into countless daily choices and opportunities.

Blood disorders have long been targets for gene therapy because their biology is relatively well understood and their cells are accessible. In conditions like beta thalassemia and sickle cell disease, mutations in the genes for hemoglobin cause red blood cells to malfunction, leading to anemia, pain, organ damage, and reduced lifespan. Standard treatment often involves repeated blood transfusions, medications, and sometimes bone marrow transplants, each with its own risks and burdens. Gene therapy takes a different approach by modifying a patient's own blood-forming stem cells. These cells are collected, edited or supplemented with a functional gene, and then returned to the body after conditioning. Over time, they give rise to new red blood cells that carry improved hemoglobin.

For many people living with these blood disorders, the prospect of a one-time procedure that could liberate them from cycles of transfusion and hospital visits is both thrilling and daunting. Clinical experiences show that some recipients of gene therapy have achieved stable levels of healthy hemoglobin and have been able to discontinue regular transfusions. Others have seen marked reductions in painful crises and improved energy for daily activities. These are not abstract metrics but tangible shifts in what life feels like from the inside. Being able to plan ahead without worrying about the next transfusion, to travel more freely, or simply to wake up with less fear of sudden pain can transform a person's relationship to their own body. At the same time, patients must weigh these potential gains against the risks of the procedure, including intensive chemotherapy to prepare the bone marrow and the unknowns of long-term effects.

Beyond replacing missing genes, gene therapy also allows for fine-tuning the behavior of cells in more subtle ways. Some approaches do not insert brand-new genes but instead increase or decrease the expression of existing ones, or introduce regulatory molecules that guide how cell pathways operate. In certain immune deficiencies, for example, a carefully calibrated boost to the activity of a crucial gene can help immune cells function more effectively without tipping them into harmful overactivity. In other cases, gene therapy may introduce a synthetic receptor that helps immune cells recognize specific targets, as in some cancer immunotherapies. These strategies treat the genome not as a static list but as a dynamic system that can be adjusted for better performance.

Real-world stories of gene therapy in cancer involve both dramatic successes and sober reminders of complexity. For some blood cancers, engineered T cells—created using gene transfer techniques—have led to deep remissions in people whose disease had resisted multiple other treatments. Patients who had exhausted standard chemotherapy options and faced grim prognoses sometimes experienced their tumors shrinking to levels that were undetectable. They could go home, reconnect with loved ones, and rebuild lives they had begun to prepare to leave. Yet these therapies can also cause intense immune reactions, and not every patient responds. Even when remissions are achieved, close follow-up is necessary to monitor for relapse or late effects. Gene-based cancer treatments thus stand as powerful but demanding tools, requiring specialized centers and careful patient selection.

Behind each success story lies the long arc of research, trial, and revision. Early gene therapy trials in the late twentieth century were marked by both promise and tragedy, including serious adverse events that shook public confidence. These experiences forced researchers, regulators, and ethicists to reevaluate how studies were designed and monitored. Safety standards were tightened, vector designs improved, and protocols became more cautious and transparent. Over time, these changes contributed to the safer, more effective therapies now reaching patients. The history is a reminder that breakthroughs often emerge not from a single triumph but from cycles of learning that include setbacks. The patients and families who participated in early trials, even when outcomes were not what they hoped, helped pave the way for those who benefit today.

Equity and access remain central concerns as gene therapy expands. Many of the most advanced treatments are among the most expensive medical interventions ever created, reflecting the complexity of their development and manufacture. Health systems must grapple with how to allocate resources, insurers must decide what to cover, and societies must debate what constitutes a fair price for potentially life-changing benefit. Some argue that high upfront costs may be offset by long-term savings if cured or substantially improved patients require fewer hospitalizations and less supportive care. Others worry that such future savings do not automatically translate into equitable access, especially for marginalized communities or countries with limited healthcare budgets. Without deliberate efforts to address these issues, gene therapy risks becoming a symbol of a divided medical future.

The logistics of delivering gene therapy also shape who can receive it. Specialized centers, trained staff, and sophisticated equipment are often needed to perform procedures and manage follow-up care. Patients may have to travel long distances, take extended time away from work or school, and navigate complex systems of authorization and reimbursement. These demands can be particularly challenging for families with fewer financial resources or caregiving support. Efforts are underway to simplify delivery methods, develop more robust outpatient protocols, and build capacity in more regions. Nevertheless, each new therapy raises the question: how can we ensure that breakthroughs written in scientific journals become options in the lives of those who need them most, regardless of post-code or income.

Gene therapy's impact is not limited to physical health; it also reshapes identities and expectations. For someone who has lived their entire life with a chronic, highly visible genetic condition, undergoing a transformative treatment can feel like stepping into a new role. They may experience a mix of relief, gratitude, survivor's guilt, or even uncertainty about how to relate to communities of others who still live with the condition. Families who have organized their daily routines around medical needs may need time to adjust to a different rhythm. Psychosocial support and honest conversations about these transitions can be as important as the biological details. Healing at the genetic level often intersects with healing at the emotional and social levels in ways that medicine is still learning how to support.

As clinicians gain more experience with gene therapies, new questions emerge about timing and patient selection. For some conditions, the best outcomes occur when treatment is given very early, before irreversible damage accumulates. This pushes medicine toward earlier diagnosis, sometimes even in newborns, and raises questions about screening programs and informed consent for families. For other conditions, waiting may allow the collection of more safety data or the development of improved techniques, but at the cost of living with ongoing disease. Patients and clinicians must weigh these trade-offs together, considering the current state of evidence and the pace of innovation. There is no single correct answer; only choices that align better or worse with each person's values and circumstances.

Looking to the future, gene therapy is likely to become more precise, more versatile, and, one hopes, more widely available. Improvements in delivery systems may allow safer targeting of specific tissues, reducing the risk of off-target effects. Refinements inspired by techniques like CRISPR may enable more exact control over where and how genetic changes occur. Manufacturing processes may become more scalable, lowering costs and simplifying logistics. At the same time, new ethical and regulatory frameworks will need to evolve to keep pace with these capabilities, protecting patients while not unduly stifling innovation. The path ahead will be shaped not only by what is technically possible but also by what societies decide is desirable and just.

In the broader context of biotechnology, gene therapies in action serve as proof that rewriting the instructions of life can move from theory to practical care. They show that conditions once considered fixed features of a person's existence can, in some cases, be altered at their roots. They remind us that behind molecular diagrams and clinical trial charts are real people whose daily lives are changed when science works as hoped. At the same time, they keep us honest about the limits of what is currently feasible, the risks that remain, and the inequality that must be confronted. As we continue through this book, gene therapy will appear again and again, intertwined with advances in stem cells, immune engineering, and aging research. Each new chapter builds on the same fundamental insight: when we can understand and adjust the code within our cells, we gain new ways to relieve suffering—and new responsibilities for how we use that power.

Chapter .6

Cellular Alchemy

Stem cells and regenerative medicine are being used to grow, repair, and replace damaged tissues.

The idea of regenerating the body has long lived at the edge of myth and medicine. Stories of miraculous healing, fountains of youth, and bodies made new again have traveled through cultures for centuries. Modern regenerative medicine does not promise immortality, but it does offer something quieter and more grounded: the possibility that certain damaged tissues might be repaired rather than merely worked around. At the center of this possibility are stem cells, the remarkably flexible cells capable of becoming many different types of tissue. By learning how to guide and harness these cells, scientists are attempting a kind of cellular alchemy—turning raw potential into specific structures that can heal. What once sounded like a fantasy is gradually being translated into clinical trials, protocols, and, in some cases, approved therapies.

Stem cells are defined less by what they are at any given moment and more by what they can become. In early development, they are like unspecialized apprentices, able to follow many possible career paths depending on the signals they receive. Some will grow into neurons that carry thoughts and sensations; others will become heart muscle cells that contract tirelessly for decades. Even in adults, small populations of stem or progenitor cells persist in tissues such as bone marrow, skin, and gut, quietly replenishing cells that wear out. The discovery and characterization of these cells gave researchers a new toolkit, one that could, in principle, be used to replace what injury or disease has taken away. The challenge lies in coaxing stem cells to grow into the right kinds of tissue, in the right place, at the right time.

A major breakthrough in this field came with the development of induced pluripotent stem cells, often abbreviated as iPSCs. Scientists learned how to take ordinary adult cells—like skin or blood cells—and reprogram them back into a stem-like state by introducing a small set of key genes. These reprogrammed cells behave much like embryonic stem cells, with the capacity to become many different cell types. This discovery sidestepped some of the ethical debates associated with using embryos and opened a door to creating patient-specific stem cells. In practical terms, it meant that a person's own cells could potentially be turned into a personalized supply of neurons, heart cells, or other tissues for study and, someday, for therapy. The body, it seemed, carried within it the instructions needed to rebuild parts of itself if we could learn how to read and apply them.

Regenerative medicine uses stem cells in several broad ways. One approach is to inject or infuse them into damaged tissues, hoping they will engraft, survive, and contribute to repair. Another approach is to grow cells or tissues outside the body and then implant them where they are needed, like crafting a biological patch. A third strategy uses stem cells primarily as factories for helpful molecules—such as growth factors—that stimulate the body's own repair processes without necessarily becoming part of the tissue themselves. Each strategy reflects a slightly different philosophy about how much rebuilding should be done by imported cells and how much by the host's own biology. In practice, many therapies blend these ideas, using transplanted cells to jump-start or guide healing that the body completes.

Blood and immune disorders were among the first areas where regenerative principles quietly entered routine practice. Bone marrow and hematopoietic stem cell transplants, used for decades to treat leukemias, lymphomas, and some genetic conditions, are essentially stem cell therapies. In these procedures, diseased or damaged blood-forming cells are replaced with healthy ones from a donor or from the patient's own previously collected cells. The new stem cells take up residence in the marrow and, if all goes well, reconstitute the entire blood and immune system. This is a powerful form of regeneration, even if it is now so well established that people sometimes forget its radically biological nature. Newer regenerative therapies build on this legacy, expanding the concept from the invisible contents of bone marrow to a broader range of organs and tissues.

The heart has become a major focal point for regenerative dreams. For most of human history, a damaged heart stayed damaged; once heart muscle cells died in a heart attack, scar tissue formed in their place and pumping capacity diminished. Unlike skin or liver, the human heart has very limited natural regenerative ability. Researchers have sought ways to change this by introducing cells that could help repair or replace the lost muscle. Early studies with various types of stem or progenitor cells produced mixed results, with some hints of benefit but also many questions about how the cells worked. Over time, evidence suggested that many injected cells did not survive long-term, but they may have secreted signals that encouraged existing heart cells and blood vessels to function better. This shifted attention toward understanding the language of these signals and how to harness them more deliberately.

More advanced efforts aim to produce actual heart muscle cells from stem cells and organize them into structures that might one day patch damaged areas. In the laboratory, scientists can grow sheets of beating cardiomyocytes derived from iPSCs and study how they contract, respond to drugs, and communicate. Creating a patch robust enough to integrate into a living heart, however, is technically challenging. It must withstand constant motion, connect electrically with surrounding tissue, and receive an adequate blood supply. Progress is being made in animal models, and small steps are moving toward human trials. Even small improvements in heart function could make a significant difference for people living with heart failure. Regenerative cardiology is still in its early days, but it illustrates both the promise and complexity of building replacement parts for the most vital of organs.

The nervous system presents its own regenerative puzzles and possibilities. Unlike many other tissues, neurons in the brain and spinal cord do not naturally regrow robustly after injury in humans. Trauma, stroke, or degenerative diseases like Parkinson's can lead to lasting deficits because lost neurons are not readily replaced. Stem cell-based approaches aim to change this reality by supplying new cells that can adopt neuronal identities and integrate into existing circuits. In Parkinson's disease, for example, research has explored transplanting dopamine-producing neurons derived from stem cells into specific regions of the brain. The hope is that these cells can restore more normal signaling and alleviate symptoms such as tremors, rigidity, and slowed movement. Early studies and trials are cautious but encouraging, suggesting that at least some functional improvement is possible.

Regeneration in the spinal cord is even more complex because of the need for long-distance connections and precise organization. Some experimental therapies use stem cells not only as potential replacements for lost neurons but also as sources of factors that modulate inflammation and support surviving cells. Others aim to provide scaffolds or bridges that help axons regrow across damaged regions. These strategies often combine biological and engineering elements, reflecting the interdisciplinary nature of regenerative medicine. While a fully restorative therapy for major spinal cord injuries remains elusive, incremental gains in movement, sensation, or autonomic function can significantly enhance quality of life. Every regained ability—a bit more hand strength, improved bladder control, a small increase in independence—can feel monumental to those living with chronic injury.

The field of tissue engineering sits at the intersection of stem cells, biomaterials, and mechanical design. Here, scientists attempt to build functional tissues and, eventually, organs outside the body using scaffolds that guide cell growth. These scaffolds can be made from synthetic polymers, natural materials like collagen, or decellularized organs that have had their own cells removed, leaving behind a kind of architectural ghost. Stem cells or other appropriate cells are seeded onto or into the scaffold and provided with nutrients, growth factors, and physical cues. Over time, they can form structures that resemble blood vessels, cartilage, skin, or other tissues. Engineered skin and simple cartilage implants have already found their way into clinical use, especially for burn care and joint repair. More complex organs, like kidneys or livers, remain long-term goals but are under active investigation.

Organoids—miniature, simplified versions of organs grown in the lab—represent another remarkable application of stem cell technology. By carefully controlling the environment around pluripotent stem cells, researchers can encourage them to self-organize into three-dimensional structures that mimic aspects of the brain, intestine, lung, or other organs. These organoids are not full replacements for real organs, but they serve as powerful models for studying development, disease, and drug responses. For instance, brain organoids derived from patients with certain genetic conditions can reveal how their neurons develop differently and how those differences might be corrected. Intestinal organoids can help test how infections or drugs affect gut lining cells. In this way, regenerative tools contribute to knowledge that may improve therapies even before direct transplantation is possible.

Regenerative medicine also intersects with the body's natural healing capacities in more subtle ways. Some therapies focus on stimulating resident stem or progenitor cells to become more active, rather than adding new cells from outside. For example, treatments for joint degeneration may use concentrated mixtures of signals, such as growth factors, derived from a patient's own blood or marrow. These injections aim to nudge local cells toward repair and reduce inflammation. The evidence for different approaches is mixed and still evolving, and not every marketed "regenerative" treatment is well supported by rigorous data. Distinguishing scientifically grounded therapies from hype is an ongoing challenge, making regulation and patient education especially important in this space.

Ethics and equity weave through regenerative medicine just as they do through other areas of biotechnology. Early debates around embryonic stem cells highlighted concerns about the moral status of embryos and the sources of research material. The advent of iPSC technology alleviated some of these issues but did not entirely remove ethical questions, especially when considering the possibility of creating advanced organoids that might possess complex properties. As therapies move toward the clinic, questions arise about who will have access, how risks and benefits are communicated, and how to prevent exploitation of vulnerable patients by unproven stem cell clinics. Clear standards, robust clinical trials, and transparent oversight are necessary to protect trust while allowing innovation to proceed.

Regenerative approaches also invite us to think differently about aging and chronic illness. If tissues can be repaired or refreshed, what does it mean to grow old. Will there be opportunities to restore function at multiple points across the lifespan, or will regenerative therapies mainly target acute injuries and specific diseases. Some researchers explore the possibility of rejuvenating certain cell populations or clearing out senescent cells that accumulate with age, blending regeneration with longevity science. These ideas are compelling but still in early stages. They raise philosophical questions about how much we should strive to extend physical youthfulness and how to balance individual desires with societal implications.

On a more personal level, regenerative medicine can shift the emotional landscape of diagnosis. Being told that a joint is "worn out," that brain damage is "permanent," or that an organ is "failing" has long carried a sense of finality. Introducing the possibility—however tentative—of repair changes the conversation. It does not mean that every problem can or will be fixed, but it allows space for imagining futures that are less constrained by irreversible loss. For some patients, this unlocks hope and motivation; for others, it may also introduce difficult decisions about whether to pursue experimental treatments. Honest communication about what is realistically possible, what is still speculative, and what risks are involved is essential to navigating these choices responsibly.

Regenerative strategies rarely act in isolation. They often dovetail with gene therapies, immunotherapies, and precise diagnostics described in other chapters. A stem cell transplant might carry a corrected gene, blending regeneration with genetic repair. An engineered tissue might be designed to resist immune rejection or deliver therapeutic molecules. Organoids tested with artificial intelligence tools could guide which regenerative approach is most likely to succeed for a given patient. This interweaving of technologies is part of what makes modern biotechnology so powerful, and also so complex to govern and understand. Medicine is no longer about a single pill or procedure, but about carefully orchestrated interventions at multiple levels of biology.

As regenerative medicine advances, it will require new kinds of partnerships between clinicians, engineers, scientists, patients, and caregivers. Surgeons may collaborate with biomaterials experts; rehabilitation specialists may work closely with stem cell researchers to optimize functional recovery after treatment. Patients' lived experiences will be crucial in defining what counts as meaningful improvement and acceptable trade-offs. Policymakers and payers will need to grapple with how to evaluate long-term benefits and costs when therapies aim to restore function across many years. These conversations will be as important as any laboratory experiment in shaping the future of cellular alchemy.

In the grand arc of this book, regenerative medicine represents a shift from only defending against disease to actively rebuilding what has been lost. It shows that biology is not solely a story of degradation and decline, but also one of renewal and plasticity. Stem cells and engineered tissues are not magic; they are tools that work within the constraints and possibilities of living systems. When used wisely, they can turn some forms of damage from permanent sentences into treatable conditions. As we move forward, we will see how these regenerative approaches intersect with the immune system, the microbiome, and even the biology of aging itself, each revealing another facet of how the body can be coaxed not simply to endure, but to repair and, in some cases, to flourish again.

Chapter .7

Training the Immune System to Heal

Immunotherapies are teaching the immune system to find and destroy threats such as cancer.

The immune system is often described as the body's army, but it is just as much a teacher, diplomat, and repair crew. For most of our lives, it works quietly in the background, recognizing threats, clearing infections, and cleaning up damaged cells without us ever noticing. When it goes wrong, the consequences can be dramatic, from cancers that slip past its surveillance to autoimmune diseases in which it mistakenly attacks the body's own tissues. For decades, medicine tried mainly to suppress the immune system when it overreacted or to support it generically when it seemed weak. Recent advances have revealed a more nuanced possibility: we can train the immune system, giving it new skills and sharper tools so it can better distinguish friend from foe. Immunotherapies embody this idea, turning our own cells and molecules into living medicines that adapt, remember, and sometimes provide long-lasting protection after a single course of treatment.

One of the clearest arenas where immune training has changed outcomes is in cancer. For many years, cancer was seen as a problem of rogue cells that had little to do with immunity, treated mainly with surgery, chemotherapy, and radiation. Careful observation, however, revealed that the immune system sometimes recognizes and attacks tumors on its own, leading to rare but striking spontaneous remissions. Researchers began to ask why the immune system usually fails to finish the job and how its natural tendencies could be encouraged rather than ignored. They discovered that tumors often hide behind molecular "brakes" on immune cells or create a toxic local environment that exhausts the body's defenders. Training the immune system to heal, in this context, means removing those brakes and restoring confidence to cells that have been tricked into standing down.

Immune checkpoint inhibitors were among the first immunotherapies to transform standard cancer care. These drugs target proteins on T cells or tumor cells that normally act as safety switches, preventing excessive immune reactions that could damage healthy tissues. Tumors exploit these switches by overactivating them, effectively telling T cells to stop attacking. Checkpoint inhibitors block that deceptive signal, allowing T cells to wake up and resume their work. For some patients with advanced melanoma, lung cancer, and other malignancies, this has led to durable remissions that persist for years after treatment ends. The idea is not to attack the tumor directly with a chemical weapon, but to remove the blindfold from the body's own soldiers and let them see their target again.

Another powerful approach, known as chimeric antigen receptor T cell therapy, or CAR-T, takes immune training to a more engineered extreme. In this process, clinicians collect a patient's T cells, modify them in the laboratory to recognize a specific marker on cancer cells, and then expand their numbers. The modified cells are infused back into the patient, where they seek out and destroy cells displaying the targeted marker. These CAR-T cells carry a synthetic receptor that functions like a custom-built sensor, combining the precision of biotechnology with the adaptability of living cells. For certain blood cancers, such as some leukemias and lymphomas, CAR-T therapies have produced dramatic responses in patients who had exhausted other options. Watching these cells expand, attack the cancer, and sometimes persist as a memory population is like witnessing a personalized immune army being trained and deployed in real time.

The very power that makes immunotherapies effective also gives rise to serious side effects in some cases. When the immune system is unleashed or augmented, it can sometimes overshoot and damage healthy organs, causing inflammation in the gut, skin, lungs, or endocrine glands. Patients receiving checkpoint inhibitors or CAR-T therapies are monitored closely for signs of such reactions, which can range from mild discomfort to life-threatening syndromes. Managing these toxicities often involves temporarily dampening the immune system with steroids or other agents, a reminder that balance remains crucial even in the era of immune activation. Clinicians must walk a careful line, encouraging a strong enough response to control the disease without tipping the body into uncontrolled inflammation. This delicate balancing act shows that training the immune system is less like flipping a switch and more like tuning an orchestra, adjusting volume and timing across many instruments.

Vaccines represent one of the oldest and most successful forms of immune training, teaching the body to recognize pathogens before they cause serious illness. Traditional vaccines expose the immune system to weakened or inactivated forms of viruses and bacteria, or to key fragments of them, prompting the development of memory cells that stand ready for future encounters. In recent years, similar principles have been applied to cancer, creating experimental vaccines that present tumor-specific proteins to the immune system. The goal is to help T cells and antibodies recognize the subtle differences that distinguish cancer cells from their healthy neighbors. Some cancer vaccines are personalized, crafted from the unique mutations found in an individual's tumor, making each dose as specific as a fingerprint. While the field is still in development, these approaches illustrate how vaccination is evolving from a population-wide shield against infection to a tailored tool for training immunity in the context of chronic disease.

Messenger RNA technologies have added a new level of flexibility to vaccine-based immune training. Instead of manufacturing proteins in factories and injecting them directly, mRNA vaccines provide cells with instructions to briefly produce selected proteins themselves. The immune system responds to these self-made proteins as if they were from an invading pathogen, building a memory response without exposure to the full virus or bacterium. Once the mRNA is degraded, the temporary factory shuts down, but the trained immune cells remain. The rapid development and deployment of mRNA vaccines against a novel virus demonstrated how quickly this platform can adapt to emerging threats. Researchers are now exploring its use for other infectious diseases, autoimmune modulation, and even some cancers, envisioning a future where immune training can be updated almost as readily as software.

Not all immune training involves making responses stronger; sometimes the goal is to teach the immune system to be less reactive toward certain targets. Autoimmune diseases like type 1 diabetes, multiple sclerosis, and rheumatoid arthritis arise when immune cells mistakenly identify parts of the body as enemies. Traditional treatments often rely on broad immunosuppression, which can reduce symptoms but also increases vulnerability to infections and other complications. Newer strategies aim to restore tolerance more selectively, educating the immune system that specific proteins or cell types should be ignored rather than attacked. Experimental therapies include nanoparticles carrying self-antigens in a context that signals "do not respond," regulatory T cell infusions designed to calm inflammation, and antigen-specific vaccines that induce peaceful coexistence instead of war. These efforts reflect a shift from simply silencing the immune system to retraining its judgment about what belongs and what does not.

Allergies offer another everyday example of immune training, though they are often experienced as a nuisance rather than a life-threatening condition. In allergic individuals, the immune system reacts strongly to harmless substances like pollen, foods, or animal dander, releasing chemicals that cause symptoms ranging from sneezing to anaphylaxis. Allergen immunotherapy, sometimes called desensitization, involves giving gradually increasing doses of the allergen over months or years. This controlled exposure can shift the immune response from an aggressive, antibody-driven reaction toward a more tolerant, regulated state. For many people, successful immunotherapy significantly reduces symptoms and the need for medications, making daily life more comfortable and safer. Though it does not rely on high-tech genetic tools, this long-practiced approach embodies the core concept of teaching the immune system to respond differently to the same stimulus.

Training the immune system also includes providing it with tools it did not generate on its own, such as monoclonal antibodies. These lab-engineered molecules are designed to bind specific targets on viruses, bacteria, or diseased cells, effectively acting as precision-guided missiles. When infused into a patient, they offer immediate, though temporary, protection or therapeutic effect, buying time while the body mounts or recalibrates its own responses. In some cases, monoclonal antibodies are used alongside vaccines, combining the quick defense of passive immunity with the durable shield of active immunity. Their design often draws on detailed knowledge of how natural antibodies work in people who have fought off infections or responded well to earlier therapies. In this way, the experiences of some immune systems can be distilled, replicated, and shared with others through biotechnology.

As with other areas of biotechnology, data and computation play a growing role in immune training. Each person's immune system carries a unique repertoire of receptors and memory cells shaped by their infections, vaccines, environment, and genetics. High-throughput sequencing now allows scientists to catalog these repertoires, creating snapshots of immune history that can be compared across individuals and time. Machine learning models analyze these patterns to predict which epitopes might make good vaccine targets, which patients are likely to respond to certain immunotherapies, and how immunity changes with age or disease. In the clinic, such tools could one day help tailor immune training plans, choosing the right combination of vaccines, cell therapies, and modulators for each person. The vision is of an immunology that is not only powerful but also personalized, treating each immune system as a distinct landscape to be mapped and cultivated.

Training the immune system to heal is ultimately about working with a living, learning network rather than imposing rigid control from outside. It acknowledges that immunity is dynamic, influenced by microbes, diet, stress, and countless other factors that medicine cannot fully dictate. By guiding and supporting this network—through vaccines, cell engineering, antibodies, and tolerance-inducing strategies—we can tilt the odds toward protection and repair. At the same time, we must remain mindful of the potential for unintended consequences when we push such a complex system in new directions. The immune system does not operate in isolation; it is in constant conversation with the trillions of microbes that inhabit our bodies and environments. In the next chapter, we will explore this unseen ecosystem, the microbiome within, and how understanding it deepens our ability to shape immunity and, ultimately, health.

Chapter .8

The Microbiome Within

The bacteria living in and on us can profoundly influence metabolism, mood, and immunity.

For much of medical history, microbes were cast as villains in the human story, invisible invaders to be killed with soap, disinfectant, and antibiotics. It is true that some bacteria and viruses cause devastating disease, and modern hygiene has saved countless lives. Yet this is only half the story, and an incomplete half at that. Inside every healthy person lives a vast, bustling ecosystem of microorganisms that are not enemies but partners. These communities, collectively called the microbiome, inhabit our gut, skin, mouth, lungs, and other surfaces, interacting constantly with our cells. To understand health in the twenty-first century, we must see ourselves not as solitary organisms, but as walking, talking collaborations between human and microbial life.

The gut microbiome is the best-studied of these ecosystems and, for good reason, often takes center stage in discussions of the microbiome. It consists of trillions of bacteria, as well as viruses, fungi, and other microscopic residents, living throughout the digestive tract, especially in the large intestine. For decades, these organisms were mostly ignored in clinical practice unless they caused obvious infection. As sequencing technologies improved, scientists began to catalog them in detail and discovered an astonishing diversity of species and genes. The genetic material of the microbiome, taken together, vastly outnumbers our human genes, offering capacities our own cells do not possess. In a sense, the microbiome acts like an extra organ, one we do not fully control but with which we are in constant conversation.

One of the microbiome's most important roles lies in digestion and metabolism. Many of the complex carbohydrates and fibers we eat cannot be broken down by human enzymes alone. Gut bacteria step in, fermenting these compounds into short-chain fatty acids and other metabolites that our cells can use for energy and signaling. This process influences how many calories we extract from food, how blood sugar is regulated, and how fat is stored. Differences in microbiome composition have been linked, in both humans and animals, to variations in weight, insulin sensitivity, and lipid profiles. While it would be an oversimplification to say that one "obese microbiome" and one "lean microbiome" exist, it is increasingly clear that our microbial partners help set the stage on which diet and genetics play out their roles.

The microbiome also helps train and modulate the immune system, especially early in life. Newborns are not born with a fully developed immune repertoire; they acquire it over time as their bodies encounter microbes from caregivers, food, and the environment. The bacteria in the gut interact with immune cells in the intestinal lining and associated lymphoid tissue, teaching them to distinguish between harmless visitors and genuine threats. When this education goes well, the immune system learns to respond appropriately, mounting defenses against pathogens while tolerating food proteins and commensal microbes. When it is disrupted—by factors like broad-spectrum antibiotics, limited microbial exposure, or certain dietary patterns—the risk of allergies, autoimmune disease, and chronic inflammation can increase. The microbiome, in this sense, acts as both a teacher and a textbook for immune development.

Signals from the microbiome do not stop at the immune system; they travel far beyond the gut. Microbial metabolites can enter the bloodstream, influencing organs such as the liver, muscles, and even the brain. Some gut bacteria produce molecules that resemble neurotransmitters or hormones, adding their voices to the chemical conversation that shapes mood, stress responses, and cognitive function. This has given rise to the concept of the "gut–brain axis," a bidirectional communication network in which the nervous system, immune system, and microbiome continually influence one another. While it is tempting to reduce this to simple claims—like "gut bacteria cause depression"—the reality is more nuanced. The microbiome is one of many factors that can tilt mental health toward resilience or vulnerability, often in combination with genetics and life experiences.

Diet is one of the most powerful levers we have to influence the microbiome. Different microbes thrive on different types of fuel, and the foods we choose act as invitations to some species and eviction notices to others. Diets rich in diverse plant fibers tend to support a more varied microbial community that produces beneficial metabolites. Diets heavy in highly processed foods, added sugars, and certain fats can, over time, favor less diverse communities that may be associated with inflammation or metabolic problems. This does not mean that a single meal will radically reshape the microbiome, but patterns over weeks and months matter. When clinicians talk about dietary changes for health, they are increasingly aware that they are not only feeding the human host but also nourishing—or neglecting—the microbial partners within.

Antibiotics add another layer of complexity to the microbiome story. These drugs have saved countless lives by eradicating dangerous infections and remain essential tools in modern medicine. At the same time, they are blunt instruments, often killing beneficial bacteria along with harmful ones. A course of broad-spectrum antibiotics can significantly reduce microbiome diversity, sometimes leading to complications like overgrowth of opportunistic pathogens in the gut. In most people, the microbiome gradually recovers, but the composition after recovery may differ from the original state. Repeated courses throughout life, especially in early childhood, may leave lasting imprints on microbial communities and health. This has led to growing calls for more judicious antibiotic use, reserving them for situations where they are clearly needed and exploring alternatives where appropriate.

Probiotics and prebiotics have entered popular conversation as ways to influence the microbiome intentionally. Probiotics are live microorganisms, often specific strains of bacteria, that are consumed in foods or supplements with the hope of conferring health benefits. Prebiotics are types of fiber or other compounds that feed beneficial microbes already present in the gut. Some probiotic products have good evidence for particular uses, such as preventing certain antibiotic-associated diarrheas or managing specific gastrointestinal conditions. However, not all products on the market are equally well studied or effective, and the benefits are often strain- and condition-specific. The idea that any generic probiotic is automatically "good for the gut" is an oversimplification, and future therapies are likely to become more targeted and personalized.

One of the most dramatic microbiome-based treatments is fecal microbiota transplantation, often abbreviated as FMT. In this procedure, stool from a carefully screened healthy donor is processed and delivered into the gut of a patient, usually through colonoscopy, capsules, or other routes. The goal is to restore a balanced microbial community in people whose microbiome has been severely disrupted, most famously in recurrent Clostridioides difficile infections that do not respond to standard antibiotics. In such cases, FMT has shown remarkable success in many patients, effectively re-seeding the gut with a community that can outcompete the pathogenic bacteria. While the idea can provoke an instinctive "yuck" reaction, for those who have lived with debilitating, recurrent infections, it can be life-changing. Ongoing research is working to refine this approach into more standardized microbial consortia and next-generation therapies.

The microbiome's influence is not confined to the gut alone; the skin microbiome also plays a vital role in health. Our skin is home to diverse communities of bacteria and fungi that help maintain barrier function, outcompete pathogens, and communicate with immune cells. Disturbances in this ecosystem have been linked to conditions such as eczema, acne, and certain infections. Traditional skincare approaches often focused solely on cleansing and sterilizing, but a newer perspective emphasizes balance rather than eradication. Emerging products and therapies aim to support or restore healthy skin microbes, using prebiotics, probiotics, or gentle formulations that avoid unnecessary disruption. As with the gut, the goal is to work with the resident ecosystem rather than wage constant war against it.

Respiratory and urogenital microbiomes are also gaining attention. The nasal passages and lungs host microbial communities that may influence susceptibility to infections and chronic conditions like asthma. The vaginal microbiome, dominated by certain beneficial Lactobacillus species in many healthy individuals, helps maintain an environment that resists infection and supports reproductive health. Disruptions, whether from antibiotics, hormonal changes, or other factors, can lead to imbalances associated with discomfort, infection, or increased risk of sexually transmitted diseases. Understanding these communities better may lead to more precise interventions, from microbiome-friendly treatments for recurrent infections to new strategies for preventing complications in pregnancy.

The relationship between the microbiome and chronic diseases extends to conditions once thought to be purely metabolic or degenerative. Research has explored links between gut microbes and cardiovascular disease, suggesting that certain microbial metabolites may contribute to atherosclerosis or blood pressure regulation. Other studies have examined associations with neurodegenerative diseases like Parkinson's and Alzheimer's, raising questions about whether microbial signals influence neuroinflammation or protein aggregation. While causality remains difficult to prove in many cases, the consistent appearance of microbiome differences in diverse conditions is hard to ignore. It suggests that the microbiome acts as a modifiable layer of biology that sits between genes, environment, and disease outcomes.

Personalized microbiome medicine envisions a future where an individual's microbial profile can guide prevention and treatment strategies. Instead of generic advice to "eat more fiber" or "avoid too many antibiotics," clinicians might review detailed microbiome analyses to suggest specific dietary changes, supplements, or interventions. A person with low diversity and particular metabolic markers might receive different recommendations than someone with a robust but imbalanced community skewed toward inflammatory species. Microbiome-based diagnostics could also help predict which patients are more likely to respond to certain drugs, including immunotherapies, since microbial metabolites can influence how the body processes medications. This is still a developing area, and robust clinical tools are only beginning to emerge, but the trajectory is clear.

Ethical and practical questions surround microbiome research and therapies as they do other forms of biotechnology. Data about a person's microbiome, like genomic information, can be deeply personal, potentially revealing aspects of diet, lifestyle, and health risks. Protecting privacy, ensuring informed consent, and preventing misuse of such data are important considerations. There is also a risk of overhyping the microbiome, turning it into a catch-all explanation for every ailment and a marketing hook for questionable products. Maintaining scientific rigor, replicating findings, and distinguishing correlation from causation are essential to avoid misleading the public. Clinicians and communicators must tread carefully, offering hopeful but honest assessments of what microbiome science can and cannot yet do.

The microbiome also forces us to reconsider what "self" means in biology. Traditional views drew a clear line between the human body and the outside world, treating microbes mostly as external actors. Microbiome science blurs that boundary, revealing a continuum of shared life whose members depend on one another. Our bodies provide habitats and nutrients; in return, microbes help digest food, train immunity, and perhaps buffer us against environmental stressors. When we change our behavior, diet, or environment, we shape not only ourselves but also our microbial communities. This interdependence challenges purely individualistic notions of health and invites more ecological thinking, where balance, diversity, and resilience matter as much inside us as they do in forests or oceans.

Biotechnology is beginning to harness the microbiome more actively, moving from observation to intervention. Engineered microbes are being developed that can sense disease-related signals in the gut and respond by producing therapeutic molecules, essentially acting as living drugs. Others might be designed to break down harmful compounds in food, neutralize toxins, or deliver vaccines at mucosal surfaces. Such applications raise new regulatory questions, because releasing modified organisms into complex ecosystems—inside and outside the body—must be done with great care. Yet the potential is enormous, offering ways to treat disease that do not rely solely on synthetic chemicals or invasive procedures. The microbiome becomes both a target and a tool in an expanding biotechnological toolkit.

On a more everyday scale, the idea of the microbiome invites us to reinterpret familiar routines through a new lens. Choices about diet, sleep, stress management, and physical activity all interact with microbial communities in subtle ways. Urban design, environmental exposures, and even social interactions influence which microbes we encounter and share. Recognizing this does not mean living in fear of every contact or obsessing over perfect microbial balance, which is neither realistic nor necessary. Instead, it suggests that caring for ourselves includes caring for the ecosystems within us, making choices that support both human and microbial well-being. In that sense, a walk in a park, a meal rich in diverse plants, or time spent in community are not only good for the mind and body, but also for the unseen companions who help keep us alive.

In the context of this book, the microbiome is a vivid example of how biotechnology has changed our understanding of what health is made of. It shows that the frontier of medicine is not only in genes and cells, but also in the communities that share our bodies and shape our biology. As we move on to organs-on-chips and living models in the next chapter, we will see how researchers are recreating aspects of these microbial and human interactions in miniature systems. These models help us experiment with complex relationships in controlled ways, bringing us closer to treatments that can restore balance rather than simply suppress symptoms. The microbiome within, once invisible and ignored, is now recognized as an essential partner in health—a partner that biotechnology is only beginning to understand and respectfully engage.

Chapter .9

Organs-on-Chips and Living Models

Miniature organ systems on chips are reinventing drug discovery and reducing reliance on animal testing.

For much of the last century, medical research relied on two main stand-ins for the human body: flat layers of cells in dishes and animals whose biology resembled ours only roughly. These models taught us an enormous amount and enabled the development of many life-saving drugs, yet they have always carried serious limitations. A single layer of cells in a plastic dish cannot reproduce the complex architecture, mechanical forces, and chemical gradients of a living organ. An animal, no matter how carefully chosen, does not share the full genetics, metabolism, or immune responses of a human being. As a result, many drugs that look promising in early testing fail in clinical trials, while some harmful side effects only emerge after a medicine is already on the market. Organs-on-chips and related living models arose from a simple but powerful question: can we build tiny, more faithful replicas of human tissues that bridge the gap between Petri dishes, animals, and real patients.

An organ-on-a-chip is not a "chip" in the sense of a silicon microprocessor, though the technologies share roots in micro-fabrication. Instead, it is a small, transparent device—often the size of a USB stick—with microscopic channels etched or molded into a flexible material. These channels can be lined with living human cells arranged to mimic the structure of a particular tissue, such as lung, liver, gut, or blood vessel. Fluids are flowed through the channels to supply nutrients and oxygen, while mechanical forces like stretching or shear stress can be applied to simulate breathing, blood flow, or peristalsis. In this way, the device becomes a kind of miniature stage on which cells experience a more lifelike environment than they ever could on a flat plastic plate. Researchers can watch them in real time under a microscope, add drugs or pathogens, and see how the "organ" responds.

One of the first widely recognized examples was the lung-on-a-chip. Engineers created a device with two parallel channels separated by a porous, flexible membrane. On one side, they grew lung epithelial cells exposed to air; on the other, they cultured blood vessel cells bathed in fluid. By rhythmically stretching the membrane, they mimicked the mechanical motion of breathing. When they introduced bacteria or nanoparticles to the air side, they could observe how the tissue barrier responded, how immune cells migrated, and how inflammation developed. In some experiments, the model reproduced key features of human lung conditions more accurately than certain animal models. This showed that it was possible to capture essential aspects of organ physiology in a device small enough to hold in one hand.

Other organ-on-chip systems soon followed. Liver chips aim to replicate the complex metabolic functions and bile flow of the liver, a crucial site for drug detoxification. Heart chips contain contracting cardiac cells that beat in synchrony, allowing researchers to measure rhythm disturbances or changes in contraction strength when exposed to new compounds. Gut chips simulate the intestinal lining, complete with mucus, flow, and, in some cases, microbial communities that interact with the epithelium. Blood–brain barrier chips model the tight junctions that protect the brain from many circulating substances, helping to identify drugs that can or cannot cross that barrier. Each platform is tuned to highlight specific aspects of physiology or disease, offering windows into processes that were previously difficult to study in controlled ways.

These devices do more than simply imitate healthy tissues; they can also model disease states. By using cells carrying particular genetic mutations, exposing tissues to damaging agents, or altering mechanical and chemical conditions, researchers can recreate elements of illnesses such as pulmonary edema, inflammatory bowel disease, fatty liver disease, or neurodegenerative disorders. In a lung chip, for example, adjusting pressure and chemical signals can reproduce the fluid leakage seen in certain acute respiratory syndromes. In a liver chip, adding high levels of fat and sugar can induce metabolic stress that resembles early liver disease. Such models allow scientists to watch the development of pathology over time, test how different interventions alter its course, and investigate why some therapies fail.

Organs-on-chips are part of a broader family of "micro-physiological systems" that also includes organoids and other three-dimensional culture models. Organoids, as described earlier, are small, self-organizing clusters of cells derived from stem cells that resemble miniature organs in structure and function. They often grow freely in a matrix rather than being constrained inside microfluidic channels. Organs-on-chips, by contrast, emphasize controlled flow, mechanical forces, and engineered architecture. The two approaches are complementary. Organoids are powerful for studying development and cell–cell communication, while chips excel at capturing interactions between tissues and circulating fluids. Increasingly, researchers are combining them—placing organoids into chip platforms to add flow and mechanical cues, yielding hybrid systems that better emulate the complexity of living organs.

One of the most compelling uses of living models is in predicting how drugs will behave in people before those drugs ever reach a human volunteer. Traditional toxicity testing relies heavily on animals and simple cell cultures, but many toxicities—especially those affecting the liver, heart, or immune system—do not appear until late in development. A liver-on-a-chip made from human cells can sometimes flag subtle toxicity at doses that would not harm a mouse, alerting drug developers earlier in the process. Similarly, a heart chip can reveal whether a new compound disrupts electrical rhythms or contraction strength, reducing the risk that a drug will later be found to cause arrhythmias. When used in panels that represent different organs, these devices can offer a more nuanced picture of safety and dose limits before moving into clinical trials.

The concept of linking multiple organ chips together to form a "body-on-a-chip" pushes this idea even further. In such systems, miniature liver, heart, kidney, gut, and other chips are connected by tiny channels through which a shared fluid circulates, carrying metabolites and drug breakdown products from one to another. This allows researchers to approximate how a drug is absorbed, modified, and cleared across the body, and how side effects in one organ may influence others. While no in vitro system can fully capture the complexity of a whole organism, these multi-organ platforms bring us closer than ever before to a controlled, human-relevant environment that can be probed, adjusted, and monitored with precision.

Organs-on-chips also play an important role in reducing reliance on animal testing. Ethical concerns, cost considerations, and scientific limitations all drive the search for alternatives that can offer better human prediction with fewer animal experiments. Regulatory agencies have begun to explore how data from well-validated chip systems could supplement or, in some contexts, partially replace animal studies in safety assessment. For this to happen at scale, chips must demonstrate reproducibility, robustness, and clear correlation with clinical outcomes. Early evidence in certain domains is promising, but broader adoption will require sustained collaboration between academic labs, industry, and regulators to build standards and share data. The ultimate goal is not simply to eliminate animal use, but to improve the quality and relevance of the information used to guide decisions about human health.

Personalization is another frontier where living models are beginning to shine. Because many organ-on-chip systems can be built using cells derived from individual patients—often through induced pluripotent stem cell technology—they can, in principle, act as "avatars" of specific people's tissues. A patient with a rare genetic heart condition, for instance, could have their cells turned into cardiac tissues on a chip. Different drugs or gene therapies could be tested on this miniature heart to see which approach restores function with the fewest side effects. Similarly, tumor-on-chip models seeded with a person's cancer cells and surrounded by supportive tissue components could be used to explore combinations of chemotherapy, targeted drugs, or immunotherapies before choosing a regimen. While still experimental, these personalized platforms hint at a future where treatment plans are informed not only by population-level data but also by direct tests on a patient's own cells.

The ecosystem around organs-on-chips is inherently interdisciplinary. Biologists bring expertise in cell behavior and tissue architecture; engineers contribute skills in micro-fabrication, fluid dynamics, and materials science; clinicians help define the most relevant questions and endpoints. Data scientists and software developers are also increasingly involved, as imaging, sensor readouts, and molecular analyses generate large datasets from each experiment. Artificial intelligence tools can assist in interpreting these data, identifying subtle patterns in cell behavior or drug responses that might escape the naked eye. In this way, living models sit at the crossroads of many of the themes in this book, embodying how biology, engineering, and computation can come together to create tools that did not exist a generation ago.

Despite their promise, organs-on-chips and related living models face significant challenges. Manufacturing devices at scale with consistent quality is technically demanding, and maintaining live, well-differentiated human cells under flow for extended periods requires careful optimization. Variability in cell sources, culture conditions, and device designs can make it difficult to compare results across labs or studies. Standardization efforts are underway, but they must balance the need for comparability with the flexibility required to tailor models to specific diseases or questions. Validation is another hurdle: for each new chip model, researchers must demonstrate that its behavior reliably mirrors key aspects of human biology and predicts outcomes in patients. This is painstaking work, but it is essential if chips are to become trusted components of regulatory and clinical decision-making.

There are also conceptual limits to what living models can capture. An organ-on-a-chip can reproduce certain mechanical and biochemical cues, but it exists in isolation from many influences present in a real body, including hormonal rhythms, full immune system complexity, and the psychological environment of stress and emotion. Organoids and chips do not think, feel, or experience the social context of illness, which means that they are tools, not surrogates for people. Even as these models become more sophisticated, they will need to be interpreted alongside data from clinical studies and patient narratives. Recognizing their strengths and constraints prevents overconfidence and helps place them appropriately in the broader landscape of medical evidence.

Ethical questions, while somewhat different from those raised by animal or human studies, still arise in the context of living models. When organoids and chips incorporate human neural tissue or begin to exhibit complex patterns of activity, some philosophers and ethicists ask whether new moral considerations come into play. Most current systems are far from any plausible threshold of consciousness or sensation, yet the trajectory of the field prompts reflection on how we will respond if models become more advanced. Issues of consent and ownership also appear, especially when cells are derived from patients for personalized chips. Clear agreements about how these cells and the data they generate can be used are important to maintain trust and respect donors' intentions.

In practical terms, the growing use of organs-on-chips and living models may change how quickly and efficiently new therapies reach patients. More predictive preclinical testing could help filter out ineffective or dangerous compounds earlier, saving time, money, and human suffering in later-stage trials. At the same time, by highlighting promising interventions with stronger evidence of human relevance, these models may accelerate the development of treatments for conditions that currently lack good options. Patients might benefit from drugs that are safer and more precisely targeted because they have already been vetted in systems that look and behave more like their own tissues. In this sense, each tiny chip in a lab has the potential to influence decisions that affect thousands or millions of lives.

In the narrative of this book, organs-on-chips and living models occupy a special place as bridges. They connect the molecular insights of genomics and gene editing with the messy reality of whole-body physiology. They offer a testing ground where regenerative therapies, immunotherapies, and microbiome-based interventions can be combined and probed in controlled ways. They also symbolize a shift in mindset: instead of accepting blunt tools and imperfect stand-ins, biotechnology increasingly seeks to build nuanced, human-relevant systems that reflect the complexity of life. As we turn next to synthetic biology and bioengineering, we will see how the same spirit of design and control is being applied at an even deeper level—creating new biological systems and components that did not arise in nature but may help solve some of medicine's hardest problems.

Chapter .10

Synthetic Biology and Bioengineering

Scientists are designing new biological systems to solve complex medical problems.

Synthetic biology begins with a bold question: what if we could design living systems the way engineers design circuits, engines, or software. Traditional biology has focused on understanding how cells and organisms already work, teasing apart pathways and mechanisms through careful observation. Synthetic biology turns that approach on its head by asking how we can build new biological parts and programs that do not exist in nature. It treats DNA as a coding language, cells as platforms, and molecules as modules that can be wired together in novel ways. The goal is not to replace natural biology, but to extend it, shaping cells to sense, compute, and act in ways that solve human problems. In medicine, this means creating living tools that can detect disease, deliver drugs, and respond intelligently to their surroundings.

At the heart of synthetic biology is the idea of biological "parts" and "circuits." Just as electronic engineers use standardized components like resistors and transistors, synthetic biologists look for genetic elements that can be combined in predictable ways. Promoters, switches, sensors, and output genes are assembled into circuits that respond to signals and carry out programmed tasks. For example, a bacterial cell might be engineered to turn on a fluorescent protein only when exposed to a specific chemical environment. Another circuit might cause cells to commit suicide if they stray outside a safe location in the body. Each design builds on a library of parts whose behavior has been measured and characterized, allowing more complex systems to be constructed layer by layer. This modular approach brings a sense of design discipline to the inherently messy world of living cells.

One of the earliest success stories in synthetic biology was the reprogramming of microbes to manufacture valuable molecules. Yeast and bacteria have been engineered to produce medicines that were once difficult or expensive to obtain from natural sources. For instance, cells can be outfitted with pathways that synthesize complex drug precursors, which are then purified and formulated into therapies. This transforms microbes into miniature factories, running on sugar and nutrients instead of steel and fossil fuels. Such microbial manufacturing can make certain drugs more affordable, reliable, and environmentally friendly. It also allows rapid adaptation if supply chains for plant- or animal-derived ingredients are disrupted. In this way, synthetic biology quietly supports medicine behind the scenes, long before patients see a pill or injection.

Beyond producing existing drugs, synthetic biology opens the door to entirely new classes of therapeutic molecules. Enzymes can be redesigned to catalyze reactions that natural enzymes never evolved to perform. Novel peptides and proteins can be crafted with properties that improve stability, specificity, or delivery. Some designs draw inspiration from nature, tweaking existing molecules to enhance their function. Others are more radical, incorporating non-standard amino acids or backbone structures that resist degradation. These custom-built biomolecules broaden the therapeutic palette available to clinicians, potentially targeting pathways that were once considered undruggable. When combined with insights from genomics and structural biology, they allow a level of precision akin to custom-tailored clothing rather than off-the-rack garments.

Synthetic biology does not stop at individual molecules; it extends to whole cells acting as smart therapeutics. Engineers have designed bacteria that can sense signals in the gut associated with inflammation and respond by secreting anti-inflammatory compounds. Other strains are being developed to detect markers of cancer or infection and release payloads only in their presence. These living medicines can, in principle, adjust their behavior in real time, responding to changing conditions in ways static drugs cannot. They can also be programmed with safety features that limit their survival outside specific environments, reducing the risk of unintended spread. The idea of swallowing or injecting engineered microbes may feel unusual at first, but it builds on the long history of using beneficial bacteria in fermented foods and probiotics, now augmented with precise genetic instructions.

Immune cells are also fertile ground for synthetic design. Building on the concept of CAR-T therapies, researchers are creating more sophisticated immune circuits that can integrate multiple signals before deciding whether to attack. For example, a T cell might be engineered to recognize two markers on a cancer cell and only become fully activated when both are present, reducing the risk of harming healthy tissue that expresses just one. Additional modules can be added to sense inflammatory cues, secrete supportive cytokines, or shut down if toxicity arises. These multi-input, multi-output designs give immune cells a kind of programmable logic, akin to tiny computers patrolling the body. As designs grow more complex, they raise both exciting possibilities and serious responsibilities for ensuring control and safety.

Bioengineering, closely intertwined with synthetic biology, focuses on building structures and systems that integrate biological components with materials and devices. In tissue engineering, for instance, scaffolds made from polymers, hydrogels, or decellularized organs are combined with cells to create functional tissues. These constructs may serve as implants, patches, or test platforms, depending on their design. Bioengineers carefully tune the stiffness, porosity, and chemical signals of scaffolds to guide how cells grow and differentiate. They also incorporate channels for nutrients, mechanical supports, and electrical cues when necessary. The result is a kind of architectural practice at the cellular scale, where form and function are inseparable, and success is measured in tissue survival, integration, and performance.

Wearable and implantable devices represent another frontier of bioengineering. Sensors that continuously monitor physiological signals—such as glucose levels, heart rhythms, or oxygen saturation—are increasingly being merged with algorithms and actuators. A closed-loop insulin pump, for example, uses sensor data to adjust hormone delivery automatically, creating an artificial pancreas that helps people with diabetes maintain more stable blood sugar. Implantable neurostimulators can modulate brain or spinal cord activity to treat pain, movement disorders, or depression. As these systems become more refined, they embody a merger of electronics and biology, where feedback loops are designed to support homeostasis. The design challenge lies not only in making the hardware reliable but also in crafting algorithms that respect the complexity and variability of human bodies.

Synthetic biology and bioengineering also intersect in the emerging field of biocompatible and bioresponsive materials. These are materials that can interact smoothly with tissues, sensing local conditions and adjusting their properties. Hydrogels might stiffen or soften in response to pH or enzymes, releasing drugs only when certain signals are present. Coatings on implants can be engineered to resist bacterial colonization while encouraging integration with bone or soft tissue. Even sutures and wound dressings can be imbued with antimicrobial properties or factors that promote healing. These innovations may seem modest compared with gene editing or cell therapies, but they can significantly reduce complications, infections, and recovery times for millions of people undergoing routine procedures.

Designing new biological systems inevitably involves risk, especially when they are intended to operate inside the body or in the environment. One core principle of responsible synthetic biology is the inclusion of safety features and "kill switches" in engineered organisms. Genetic circuits can be built so that cells require specific nutrients or conditions only found in controlled settings, making it difficult for them to survive elsewhere. Other safeguards include self-destruct mechanisms that activate after a certain number of cell divisions or in response to unplanned signals. These measures are not foolproof, but they demonstrate an ethic of anticipating failure modes and building in layers of protection. As designs become more powerful, the importance of rigorous risk assessment and transparent oversight only grows.

Ethical questions in synthetic biology go beyond safety to touch on deeper issues of purpose and values. When we design new biological functions, what goals should guide our efforts, and who gets to decide. Some people worry that synthetic biology represents an attempt to "play God," altering life in ways that disrespect natural boundaries. Others view it as a continuation of humanity's long history of cultivating, breeding, and modifying organisms for food, medicine, and companionship. The key differences now are the speed, precision, and scale at which changes can be made. Inclusive public dialogue, shaped by diverse cultural and philosophical perspectives, is essential to ensure that synthetic biology is directed toward widely shared benefits, not narrow interests.

Economic and social implications also loom large. If engineered microbes can produce drugs cheaply in fermenters, how will this affect farmers who grow medicinal plants or workers in conventional manufacturing. When living medicines and complex bioengineered devices become standard, will their cost limit access to wealthy health systems, or will they be made broadly affordable. Intellectual property systems will influence who can build on existing designs and who profits from successful applications. There is a risk that synthetic biology could deepen inequities if its benefits cluster in already advantaged communities. At the same time, if managed with justice in mind, it could lower costs, decentralize production, and increase resilience of medical supply chains worldwide. The outcome is not predetermined; it will emerge from policy choices and collective priorities.

Education and transparency are crucial to building trust as synthetic biology moves from labs into clinics and communities. Patients need clear explanations when treatments involve engineered cells, microbes, or materials, including what is known, what remains uncertain, and how risks are being managed. Communities asked to host biomanufacturing facilities or research centers deserve information about environmental controls and safety protocols. Scientists and engineers have a responsibility to communicate not just successes but also setbacks and limitations, resisting hype and acknowledging uncertainties. In doing so, they invite the public into a shared project of shaping how these tools are used, rather than presenting finished products as fait accompli.

Synthetic biology and bioengineering also offer new ways to engage with global challenges that intersect with health, such as climate change and pollution. Organisms can be engineered to break down environmental toxins, capture carbon, or produce sustainable alternatives to petrochemicals. These efforts can indirectly improve health by reducing air and water pollution, mitigating climate-related disasters, and securing food supplies. At the same time, releasing engineered organisms into open environments requires careful ecological evaluation, robust monitoring, and international cooperation. The line between medical and environmental biotechnology is increasingly porous, reminding us that human health is inseparable from the health of the planet.

On a personal level, synthetic biology invites a shift in how we think about our bodies and medicines. Treatments may increasingly resemble collaborations between human systems and designed biological helpers, rather than one-directional interventions. A person with a chronic illness might host a community of engineered microbes tuned to support their physiology, while wearing devices that listen to their body and adjust therapies automatically. An implanted scaffold could slowly dissolve as new tissue grows in its place, leaving behind no foreign hardware. These scenarios are not science fiction; they are sketches of projects already underway. They hint at a future where medicine feels less like a series of external shocks and more like a guided conversation between designed and natural processes.

In the context of this book, synthetic biology and bioengineering represent the creative frontier of biotechnology. They show how deeply we are beginning to understand and shape the rules by which living systems operate. This power carries obvious risks, but it also opens doors to solutions for diseases and challenges that have long resisted conventional approaches. When combined with genomics, gene therapies, regenerative strategies, and immune training, synthetic biology becomes part of a broader toolkit for rewriting what is possible in health care. As we move next to artificial intelligence as a lab partner, we will see how digital tools amplify this creative capacity, helping to design, simulate, and optimize biological systems before they ever touch a cell.

Author Reflection – Synthetic Biology and Bioengineering

Writing about synthetic biology, I felt the tension between awe and caution more strongly than almost anywhere else in this book. There is something breathtaking about watching living cells carry out tasks we designed on a computer screen, like seeing ideas made flesh. At the same time, I am acutely aware that every new capability arrives in a world that is already unequal, fragile, and full of unintended consequences. The question that stays with me is not "Can we build this," but "Should we, and under what conditions." I am encouraged by the many scientists, engineers, and community advocates who are trying to build a culture of responsibility around this work, not as an afterthought but as part of the design process itself. My hope is that readers come away not only impressed by what is possible, but also inspired to participate in the conversations that will decide how these possibilities are used.

Inspirational Quotes

Designing with life is not an excuse to control it, but an invitation to collaborate with it more wisely.

Chapter .11

AI as a Lab Partner

Artificial intelligence is accelerating drug discovery and diagnosis and treatment planning.

For most of the history of medicine, discovery has depended on human eyes, human intuition, and human patience. Scientists sifted through data by hand, sketched curves on paper, and trusted their hunches when patterns seemed to emerge. Clinicians learned to recognize subtle shadows on X-rays or faint murmurs in a stethoscope through years of experience and repetition. Today, those human skills are being joined by another kind of helper: artificial intelligence systems that can see patterns in data too vast or too complex for any single person to grasp. These systems are not replacements for curiosity or judgment, but amplifiers that can sort, compare, and predict at extraordinary speed. When they are thoughtfully integrated, they become lab partners and clinical allies rather than distant, inscrutable machines.

In the laboratory, artificial intelligence has become a powerful engine for identifying new drug candidates. Traditional drug discovery often involved testing huge libraries of molecules in wet labs, hoping that a few would interact with a target in the right way. Now, machine learning models can analyze the shapes of proteins, the chemistry of known drugs, and the features of successful therapies to propose new compounds in silico. Generative algorithms can design molecules that fit a target like a key in a lock, then predict properties such as solubility or toxicity before a single synthesis step is taken. This narrows the field, allowing chemists to focus their efforts on the most promising ideas. In effect, AI helps scientists search a nearly infinite chemical space with far greater efficiency than random trial and error.

Artificial intelligence also helps interpret the flood of biological data streaming from modern experiments. Genomics, proteomics, metabolomics, and other "omics" approaches produce high-dimensional datasets that capture thousands of variables per sample. Human researchers can see only so much when staring at spreadsheets or static plots, no matter how skilled they are. Machine learning methods, especially those designed for complex pattern recognition, can find clusters, trajectories, and relationships that would otherwise remain hidden. They can identify combinations of gene expression changes that predict drug response or disease progression, even when no single marker stands out. These insights provide hypotheses that can be tested in the lab, turning AI from a black box into a generator of concrete, testable ideas.

One of the most dramatic demonstrations of AI's scientific power has been in predicting protein structure. For decades, determining how a protein's chain of amino acids folds into a three-dimensional shape required painstaking experimental work. Misfolding and subtle conformational changes can mean the difference between health and disease, so structural biology has always been central to drug design. Advanced AI models trained on known structures have learned to infer the likely shapes of many proteins directly from their sequences. This does not replace experimental confirmation, but it gives researchers a head start and a framework for understanding how proteins interact. In turn, that understanding guides the design of drugs that bind more specifically and effectively.

Beyond analysis and prediction, AI is increasingly embodied in "self-driving labs." In these setups, robotic systems perform experiments under the guidance of algorithms that decide what to test next. The AI analyzes results in near real time, updates its models, and selects the most informative next step, much like a scientist iteratively refining their approach. This can dramatically accelerate tasks such as optimizing reaction conditions, searching for new materials, or screening biological pathways. The human role shifts from manually running every experiment to designing goals, constraints, and safety checks for the automated system. Rather than replacing scientists, self-driving labs free them to focus on conceptual questions, interpretation, and creativity while their robotic partners handle repetitive work.

On the clinical side, AI has made some of its earliest marks in fields that rely heavily on imaging. Radiology, pathology, and dermatology all involve interpreting visual patterns, making them natural arenas for computer vision systems. Deep learning models can be trained on large collections of labeled images to recognize features associated with tumors, fractures, infections, or inflammatory conditions. In some controlled studies, these systems have matched or even exceeded human experts on specific tasks, such as spotting tiny lung nodules or early diabetic changes in the retina. In practice, they are best used as second readers, highlighting areas of concern and reducing the risk of oversight. The goal is not to replace radiologists or pathologists, but to give them another set of eyes that never tire and never lose focus.

Artificial intelligence is also being used to make sense of the often chaotic information in electronic health records. Clinical notes, lab results, medication lists, and imaging reports accumulate over years, creating a dense history that can be hard to digest during a short appointment. Natural language processing tools can extract key facts from free-text notes, flag potential drug interactions, and surface trends that might otherwise be missed. Predictive models can estimate the likelihood of events like hospital readmission, sepsis, or cardiac arrest based on subtle combinations of vital signs and lab values. When integrated thoughtfully, these systems can nudge clinicians to pay attention to patients at rising risk, supporting earlier intervention. The challenge lies in presenting these insights clearly and avoiding alarm fatigue rather than overwhelming clinicians with constant alerts.

Treatment planning is another domain where AI's pattern-recognition abilities can support decision-making. For complex conditions like cancer or heart failure, there are often many possible treatment pathways, each with its own probabilities of benefit and harm. Machine learning models trained on large datasets of past patients can suggest which combinations of therapies tended to work best for those with similar profiles. They can account for factors such as age, comorbidities, genetic variants, and previous responses to treatment. These recommendations are not prescriptive orders; they are additional inputs alongside clinical guidelines and patient preferences. Ideally, they help clinicians have more informed, individualized conversations rather than relying solely on population averages or personal anecdote.

AI-powered tools are also reaching patients more directly through digital health applications. Smartphone apps and wearables can collect continuous streams of data on heart rate, activity, sleep, and sometimes even heart rhythms or glucose levels. Algorithms sift through this data to detect trends, anomalies, or patterns that correlate with flares of disease or deteriorations in health. A patient with chronic heart failure might receive a prompt if subtle changes suggest fluid buildup, encouraging them to contact their care team before symptoms become severe. Someone with diabetes might get real-time feedback on how different foods or exercises affect their glucose, learning over time how to adjust. In these cases, AI acts like a background coach, offering gentle course corrections based on patterns too subtle or tedious for humans to track alone.

With all its promise, AI in medicine also brings serious risks and limitations that cannot be ignored. The quality of an algorithm's output depends heavily on the data used to train it, and medical data often reflect existing biases and inequities. If a model is trained primarily on records from one demographic group, it may perform poorly for others, potentially worsening disparities in diagnosis or treatment. Even when performance metrics look impressive overall, errors can cluster in ways that harm marginalized populations. Addressing these issues requires careful dataset curation, ongoing auditing, and a commitment to fairness as a design objective rather than an afterthought. It also demands transparency about where models are likely to be less reliable, so clinicians do not over-trust them in inappropriate contexts.

Interpretability is another major concern. Many of the most powerful AI models, especially deep neural networks, operate in ways that are difficult for humans to fully understand. In medicine, where decisions can have profound consequences, clinicians and patients often want to know why a certain recommendation was made. Explainable AI techniques aim to shed light on which features or patterns contributed most to a prediction, offering heat maps on images or highlighting key variables in tabular data. While these explanations are not perfect windows into the model's inner workings, they provide useful clues and starting points for human judgment. Over time, the dialogue between interpretable insights and clinical expertise may help refine both the models and the practice of medicine itself.

Privacy and security loom large whenever personal health data and powerful algorithms meet. Training robust AI systems often requires large datasets that include sensitive information about diagnoses, treatments, and outcomes. Protecting this data from misuse or breaches is a technical and ethical imperative. Techniques such as de-identification, secure multi-party computation, and federated learning—where models are trained across decentralized data without centralizing raw records—offer promising paths forward. Yet technology alone is not enough; clear governance, consent processes, and accountability frameworks are essential. Patients need to know who can access their data, for what purposes, and how they can exercise control over its use.

In the clinical setting, responsibility for decisions must remain clearly grounded in human professionals, even when AI tools are involved. A model may suggest that a scan shows malignancy or that a patient is at high risk of deterioration, but it is clinicians who integrate this with physical examination, patient history, and values. They must be able to accept or reject AI recommendations, document their reasoning, and be accountable for outcomes. This human-in-the-loop approach recognizes that algorithms can be wrong, incomplete, or misapplied. It also respects the importance of empathy, communication, and ethics in medicine—dimensions where AI has no independent capacity. Building systems that support, rather than erode, professional autonomy is crucial to real-world adoption and trust.

Training and education will shape how effectively clinicians and scientists use AI as a lab partner. Medical and scientific curricula increasingly need to include basic literacy in data science, algorithmic thinking, and the strengths and weaknesses of machine learning. Clinicians do not need to become programmers, but they should understand enough to ask critical questions about model validation, generalizability, and bias. Similarly, data scientists working in healthcare benefit from exposure to clinical realities, including the messy, missing, and sometimes contradictory nature of real-world data. Shared language and mutual respect between these groups can turn potential friction into creative collaboration, where each side understands what the other can and cannot do.

Global equity is a recurring theme in discussions about AI in medicine. High-quality datasets, computing infrastructure, and technical expertise are often concentrated in wealthier regions and institutions. If models are developed mainly in these contexts, they may be ill-suited for settings with different disease patterns, resource constraints, or cultural practices. At the same time, AI has the potential to extend expertise into areas with shortages of specialists, offering decision support in remote clinics or underserved urban centers. Realizing this potential requires deliberate efforts to include diverse populations in data collection, to build tools adapted to low-resource settings, and to share benefits rather than hoard them. Otherwise, the AI revolution in medicine risks becoming another force that widens the gap between those with access and those without.

Looking ahead, AI is likely to become more deeply woven into every stage of biomedical innovation and care. Models will increasingly integrate multiple types of data at once—images, genomic sequences, clinical notes, sensor readings—to create richer, more holistic representations of health and disease. Drug discovery pipelines may rely on AI to generate hypotheses, plan experiments, and interpret outcomes in seamless cycles. Clinical decision support tools may become more conversational and context-aware, helping clinicians and patients explore options together rather than simply issuing static recommendations. Throughout this evolution, the core question will remain: how do we design these systems so that they enhance human dignity, agency, and safety.

In the broader story of biotechnology, artificial intelligence is less a separate character and more a set of lenses and instruments that sharpen our view. It makes it easier to see patterns in the genome, to design gene therapies and synthetic circuits, to understand regenerative processes, and to track outcomes in real-world populations. Yet its presence also forces us to confront issues of trust, transparency, and justice with new urgency. As we move into the next chapter, focused on smart diagnostics and wearable health technologies, we will see how AI leaves the confines of the lab and server room to accompany people in their daily lives. The challenge will be to ensure that this companionship serves genuine well-being rather than becoming just another source of noise, anxiety, or inequity.

Chapter .12

Smart Diagnostics and Wearable Health

Wearable devices and smart diagnostics enable continuous monitoring and early detection of disease.

For most of medical history, health care has been episodic. You felt unwell, made an appointment, sat in a waiting room, and the doctor caught a brief snapshot of your body at that moment. Between visits, medicine was largely blind. Blood pressure could spike, heart rhythms could stutter, blood sugar could swing wildly, and no one would see it unless the timing happened to line up with a clinic visit. Smart diagnostics and wearable health technologies are changing that by turning occasional snapshots into near-continuous streams. Sensors on our wrists, fingers, and even in our clothing quietly collect data as we go about daily life. When interpreted well, these signals can reveal early signs of trouble, track responses to treatment, and sometimes prevent emergencies before they fully unfold.

The modern wave of wearables began with simple activity trackers that counted steps and estimated calories burned. At first, they were seen mostly as lifestyle gadgets, more about motivation than medicine. Over time, their sensors became more capable, measuring heart rate, sleep patterns, and, in some devices, oxygen saturation and heart rhythm. This evolution blurred the line between consumer electronics and medical tools. A jogger checking their pace on a morning run might also be gathering data that, one day, helps a doctor understand fatigue or palpitations. As these devices grew more common, clinicians and researchers realized they were sitting on an enormous, largely untapped source of health information—data about how bodies behave not just in exam rooms, but in grocery lines, meetings, and dreams.

Heart health has been one of the earliest beneficiaries of wearable monitoring. Some smartwatches and patches can record electrocardiograms (ECGs) or detect irregular heart rhythms suggestive of atrial fibrillation, a condition that increases the risk of stroke. People who once experienced occasional, fleeting palpitations with no clear explanation can now capture their heart rhythm at the moment symptoms occur. Algorithms analyze these tracings and flag patterns that warrant a closer look. In some cases, wearables have alerted individuals to arrhythmias they did not even feel, prompting timely evaluation and treatment. This does not replace traditional cardiology, but it adds a new layer of vigilance that accompanies people beyond hospital walls.

Continuous glucose monitors (CGMs) are another powerful example of smart diagnostics moving into everyday life. For people living with diabetes, checking blood sugar used to mean finger-stick tests a few times a day—a sparse sampling of a constantly changing signal. CGMs use tiny sensors inserted under the skin to measure glucose in the interstitial fluid every few minutes, feeding data to a receiver or smartphone. Users can see trends in real time, learn how meals and exercise affect their levels, and receive alerts when values drift dangerously high or low. Some systems integrate with insulin pumps to automatically adjust dosing, creating partial "closed loops" that reduce the burden of constant decision-making. The combination of continuous sensing, smart algorithms, and responsive devices turns a once-punishing routine into a more manageable conversation between body and technology.

Sleep, long recognized as vital but poorly measured, has also come into clearer focus thanks to wearables. Devices that track movement, heart rate, and sometimes breathing patterns can estimate sleep duration and stages across many nights. While consumer sleep metrics are not perfect clinical tools, they give people a sense of how consistent—or inconsistent—their rest really is. Over weeks, patterns emerge: bedtimes creep later, sleep becomes more fragmented during periods of stress, or weekends diverge sharply from weekdays. Clinicians can use this information as a starting point for discussing insomnia, sleep apnea, or mood disorders. In some cases, more specialized devices that measure airflow, oxygen levels, and snoring can support the diagnosis of sleep-disordered breathing without requiring a full overnight study in a lab.

Smart diagnostics are not limited to devices worn on the body; they also include tests that can be done quickly at home or in community settings. Point-of-care tests—small kits that detect infections, measure biomarkers, or analyze samples in minutes—are becoming more sensitive and easier to use. Where once you needed to visit a clinic, wait in line for a blood draw, and wait days for results, many basic assessments can now be done on the spot. Some tests use a drop of blood from a finger prick to measure markers of inflammation, cholesterol, or organ function. Others use saliva, breath, or urine to detect infections or metabolic changes. When paired with smartphone cameras and apps that interpret results, these tools bring elements of the lab into kitchens, schools, and pharmacies.

Imaging, too, is becoming more portable and smart. Handheld ultrasound devices connect to tablets or phones, allowing clinicians to look beneath the skin at the bedside or in the field. Artificial intelligence can guide novice users toward good image capture and highlight areas of concern, making ultrasound more accessible beyond specialized departments. In the future, similar miniaturization and AI assistance may extend to other modalities, such as basic retinal imaging or lung assessment. The impact is especially significant in remote or resource-limited settings, where traditional imaging equipment is scarce. Smart diagnostics can act as force multipliers, extending the reach of expert interpretation through algorithms and telemedicine connections.

One of the most intriguing developments is the shift from reactive to proactive care. In a reactive model, tests are ordered when something seems wrong—a lump appears, pain worsens, or lab results from a routine checkup come back abnormal. In a data-rich environment, algorithms can watch for subtle changes that precede overt symptoms: a gradual increase in resting heart rate, a decline in step count and sleep quality, or repeated small spikes in blood pressure. Individually, any one of these might be dismissed as noise. Taken together over weeks or months, they can signal rising risk for depression, infection, heart failure exacerbation, or other conditions. Smart diagnostics can then trigger gentle prompts—asking how a person is feeling, suggesting a check-in with a clinician, or recommending adjustments to medication.

Of course, more data is not automatically better. Streams of numbers and alerts can easily become overwhelming or anxiety-provoking. One challenge for designers of wearables and smart diagnostics is deciding which data to show, when to show it, and how to frame it in ways that support, rather than undermine, well-being. Constant notifications about minor fluctuations can make healthy people feel fragile, fixating on variations that have no real clinical meaning. Clinicians, too, can be buried in dashboards and graphs that offer little actionable insight. The most effective systems are selective, highlighting trends that truly matter and allowing users to customize thresholds and focus areas. They turn raw data into digestible stories about health, not endless noise.

Privacy and security loom large in discussions about wearable health. Devices often collect intimate information about heart rhythms, sleep, movement patterns, and sometimes location. This data may pass through multiple companies and cloud services before being summarized for users or shared with clinicians. Safeguarding it from misuse, breaches, or surveillance is both a technical and ethical imperative. People need clear information about who can access their data, how it will be used, and how long it will be stored. Regulations and standards are evolving, but technology often moves faster than law. Trust in smart diagnostics depends not just on their accuracy, but also on confidence that they will not be turned into tools of exploitation or discrimination.

Equity is another critical consideration. Many wearables and smart devices are marketed to relatively affluent, tech-savvy consumers. Their design often assumes access to smartphones, reliable internet, and time to learn interfaces. If we are not careful, this can create a "health data divide," where some people benefit from early detection and personalized insights while others are left out. Addressing this requires deliberate effort: designing affordable devices, supporting offline or low-bandwidth modes, and integrating smart diagnostics into public health and community care programs. Clinics serving marginalized populations can be equipped with shared devices and staff trained to interpret data collaboratively with patients. Smart diagnostics should be seen as tools to narrow gaps in health outcomes, not widen them.

Smart tests and wearables also reshape the doctor–patient relationship. When people arrive at appointments with weeks of heart rate, sleep, and symptom logs on their phones, conversations change. Instead of relying solely on retrospective recall—"I think I've been more tired lately"—they can point to concrete trends. Clinicians can use this information to tailor questions, treatments, and follow-up plans. At the same time, there can be tension if data is interpreted differently by patients and providers, or if clinicians feel pressured to review more information than they realistically have time for. Establishing clear expectations about how data will be used, how often it will be reviewed, and which signals should trigger outreach is key to making these tools sustainable and supportive.

Another frontier in smart diagnostics is personalization. Just as precision medicine tailors treatment based on genetics and biology, adaptive algorithms can learn what "normal" looks like for each individual and detect deviations more accurately. A resting heart rate of ninety beats per minute might be concerning for one person and typical for another. Sleep patterns that look erratic on a generic chart may, for a particular shift worker, be entirely healthy. Personal baselines allow alerts to be calibrated to meaningful changes rather than rigid cutoffs. Over time, systems can refine their models as they observe more data, becoming better attuned to the rhythms of the person wearing them.

Smart diagnostics are also starting to incorporate context beyond biology. Mood tracking apps, digital diaries, and environmental sensors can be linked with physiological data to paint a richer picture of health. For example, correlations between air quality and asthma flares, or between social isolation and changes in sleep and activity, can emerge. This does not mean that devices should intrude into every corner of life, but it acknowledges that bodies do not exist in isolation from surroundings and experiences. When used with consent and care, contextual data helps clinicians and patients connect the dots between daily realities and physical symptoms, leading to more holistic care plans.

Regulation of smart diagnostics walks a delicate line between encouraging innovation and protecting users. Some tools clearly function as medical devices and must meet rigorous standards for safety and effectiveness. Others are marketed as wellness or lifestyle products, sitting in a gray area with fewer formal requirements. The boundary is not always clear. A heart rate monitor used for fitness may become a de facto medical device when people rely on it to detect arrhythmias. Regulators are increasingly looking at not just what a device claims to do, but how people actually use it, to determine appropriate oversight. Transparent labeling, clear communication of limitations, and ongoing post-market surveillance will all play roles in keeping smart diagnostics safe and honest.

Despite the challenges, the potential benefits of smart diagnostics and wearable health technologies are substantial. Early detection of emerging problems can mean the difference between a minor adjustment and a major crisis. Continuous data can validate the impact of lifestyle changes, medications, or therapies, giving people real-time feedback that reinforces positive habits. For those living with chronic illnesses, knowing that their body is being watched in helpful ways can bring a sense of companionship and safety—not the false security of perfection, but the reassurance that they are not navigating their condition alone. When designed and deployed thoughtfully, these tools can make health care feel less like a series of disconnected episodes and more like an ongoing relationship.

In the broader story of this book, smart diagnostics and wearable health represent medicine's shift from the clinic to the everyday. They show how advances in sensors, connectivity, and algorithms can turn ordinary objects into partners in care, from watches and phones to home tests and portable scanners. They also raise profound questions about data, trust, and what it means to live in a body that is increasingly quantified. As we move into the next chapter—focused on editing aging itself—we will see how continuous monitoring and early detection may intersect with efforts to slow or reverse aspects of biological aging. The tools that watch us grow older may eventually help us grow older differently, with more years lived in health rather than in decline.

Chapter .13

Editing Aging Itself

Longevity science and new therapies aim to extend not just lifespan but also healthspan.

For most of human history, aging was seen as an unchangeable backdrop to life, as inevitable as sunrise and tide. People focused on surviving infections, accidents, and childbirth, rarely living long enough for chronic diseases of age to dominate. As public health improved and lifespans lengthened, the landscape shifted. Heart disease, cancer, dementia, and frailty emerged as the main threats to health, clustered in the later decades of life. Medicine responded by treating each disease separately: blood pressure pills for the heart, chemotherapy for cancer, cognitive enhancers for memory. Longevity science starts from a different question: what if many of these conditions share common roots in the biology of aging itself. If so, then targeting aging processes might prevent or delay multiple diseases at once, improving not just how long we live, but how well.

Biologists often describe aging as the gradual accumulation of cellular and molecular damage. Over time, DNA acquires mutations, proteins misfold and clump, mitochondria lose efficiency, and communication between cells becomes garbled. Tissues stiffen, stem cells tire, and the immune system becomes less responsive to threats while more prone to chronic inflammation. These changes do not unfold on a fixed schedule;

lifestyle, environment, and genetics all influence the tempo. Still, certain patterns appear across many organisms, from worms to mice to humans. Longevity research seeks to understand these patterns, sometimes called "hallmarks of aging," and to identify interventions that slow or partially reverse them. The hope is that by addressing the roots of decline, we can compress the period of disability at the end of life, shifting the balance toward more years of vigor.

One of the earliest clues that aging might be malleable came from studies in simple organisms. In worms and flies, single gene mutations were discovered that significantly extended lifespan, sometimes doubling it. These genes often affected nutrient-sensing pathways that regulate how cells respond to food availability, such as insulin signaling and a protein complex known as mTOR. Reducing the activity of these pathways in model organisms tended to slow growth and reproduction but extend the period of functional life. Caloric restriction—carefully reducing calorie intake without malnutrition—produced similar effects in many species, increasing lifespan and delaying age-related diseases. These findings suggested that aging is not just random wear and tear, but a regulated process that can be tuned.

Translating these insights to humans is complex. Lifespans are long, environments varied, and ethical constraints prevent experiments as simple as those in worms or mice. Nevertheless, researchers have identified molecules in animals that mimic some of the effects of caloric restriction by targeting nutrient-sensing pathways. Drugs that inhibit mTOR, activate certain sirtuin enzymes, or influence cellular energy sensors like AMPK have extended lifespan and healthspan in several models. In humans, some of these compounds are already used for other indications, such as transplant rejection or diabetes, and are being studied for their potential to influence aging-related outcomes. The idea is not to freeze people in time, but to shift cellular priorities from short-term growth and reproduction toward long-term maintenance and repair.

Another major theme in aging biology is the role of senescent cells. These are cells that have stopped dividing in response to damage or stress but refuse to die, lingering in tissues and secreting a cocktail of inflammatory and tissue-altering molecules. In youth, senescence can be protective, preventing damaged cells from turning cancerous and supporting wound healing. With age, however, senescent cells accumulate and become a kind of molecular noise that disrupts tissue function. In mice, selectively removing these "zombie" cells has been shown to delay the onset of age-related diseases, improve physical function, and extend healthy lifespan. Drugs designed to clear senescent cells, often called senolytics, are now being tested in humans for conditions ranging from fibrotic lung disease to frailty and osteoarthritis.

Mitochondria, the tiny powerhouses inside cells, are also central to aging. They generate the energy that fuels cellular processes, but in doing so, they can produce reactive molecules that damage DNA, proteins, and lipids. Over time, mitochondrial DNA accumulates mutations, and the balance between energy production and damage control shifts unfavorably. Interventions that improve mitochondrial function or boost the cell's ability to recycle damaged components—through processes like mitophagy and autophagy—have shown promise in animal models. Some candidate therapies aim to enhance these cleanup systems, helping cells maintain a younger metabolic profile. Others explore ways to supplement or replace damaged mitochondria, though this remains technically challenging. In essence, these strategies treat cellular energy systems as maintainable infrastructure rather than disposable batteries.

The immune system, too, undergoes aging, a phenomenon sometimes called immunosenescence. As years pass, the repertoire of naïve T and B cells that can respond to new threats shrinks, while memory cells accumulate from past infections. The ability to mount vigorous responses to vaccines and pathogens declines, and chronic low-grade inflammation—dubbed "inflammaging"—rises. This state contributes to atherosclerosis, diabetes, neurodegeneration, and other conditions. Longevity science explores ways to rejuvenate immune function, from thymus-supporting therapies that help produce new T cells to strategies that rebalance inflammatory signaling. Some approaches involve cellular therapies, others small molecules or lifestyle interventions. The goal is to restore a more youthful balance between defense and restraint, enabling older bodies to respond robustly without tipping into damaging overreaction.

Telomeres, the protective caps at the ends of chromosomes, have long fascinated aging researchers. Each time a cell divides, telomeres tend to shorten slightly, and when they become critically short, the cell may enter senescence or die. This process acts as a kind of division counter, limiting how many times some cells can replicate. Shortened telomeres have been associated with increased risk of many age-related diseases, though they are only one piece of a complex puzzle. Experimental strategies to extend telomeres or enhance the activity of the enzyme telomerase have shown rejuvenating effects in certain cell types and animal models. However, because unrestrained telomerase activity can also promote cancer, any therapy aimed at telomeres must navigate a narrow path between regeneration and tumor risk. This tension exemplifies the broader challenge of editing aging: many mechanisms that keep us young also protect against cancer when constrained.

Longevity science interacts deeply with lifestyle factors, even as it explores advanced therapies. Regular movement, varied nutrient-dense diets, sufficient sleep, stress management, and social connection all influence the biology of aging at multiple levels. They affect hormone levels, inflammation, mitochondrial function, and even epigenetic marks on DNA. Some researchers argue that these behaviors are the most powerful "anti-aging interventions" we currently have, accessible to many without specialized technology. From this perspective, drugs and high-tech therapies are seen as complements, not substitutes, for supportive daily habits. At the same time, acknowledging the importance of lifestyle does not erase structural barriers that make healthy choices harder for many, such as poverty, unsafe neighborhoods, and inequitable access to care and nutritious food.

Epigenetics, the set of chemical modifications that influence gene expression without changing DNA sequence, has become a key focus in discussions of aging. With age, epigenetic patterns drift, affecting which genes are active in different tissues. Some researchers have identified "epigenetic clocks," combinations of DNA methylation marks that correlate strongly with chronological age and, in some studies, with health status and mortality risk. These clocks offer a way to measure biological age—the functional state of tissues—rather than just years lived. Intriguingly, certain interventions in animals, including reprogramming cells toward a more youthful state, can reset aspects of these epigenetic clocks. Whether safe, partial reprogramming could one day rejuvenate tissues in humans is an open question, under active investigation. It raises both exciting prospects and serious concerns about cancer risk and loss of cellular identity.

Gene editing tools, such as those described in earlier chapters, also intersect with aging research. Some age-related diseases are driven by specific genetic variants that might be amenable to correction, reducing the burden of those conditions in later life. More broadly, as we understand which genes and pathways modulate longevity in model organisms, there is temptation to consider genetic tweaks that mimic long-lived variants in humans. At present, such interventions remain hypothetical and ethically contentious, especially when they would affect germline cells and future generations. Still, the very fact that these possibilities are technically imaginable underscores how far biotechnology has moved the conversation from "aging is inevitable" to "which aspects of aging, if any, should we try to alter, and how."

Societal and ethical questions loom large when we contemplate editing aging itself. If therapies emerge that significantly extend healthspan, who will have access to them. Will they be limited to those who can pay high prices, creating an even wider gap between the health trajectories of rich and poor. How will pension systems, employment, family structures, and intergenerational relationships adapt if more people live well into their nineties or beyond. Some worry about overcrowding and resource strain, while others note that healthier older adults can contribute economically and socially longer, offsetting some burdens. The answers depend on policy choices, cultural values, and how equitably the fruits of longevity research are distributed, not on biology alone.

There is also a risk that an intense focus on extending life could overshadow efforts to improve the quality of life at any age. The pursuit of youth can drift into obsession, fueling industries that promise miracles without evidence and prey on understandable fears. Longevity science must distinguish itself from superficial anti-aging fads by grounding claims in rigorous data and acknowledging limits. Compassionate care for older adults includes respect for the natural arc of life, including its final chapters, even as we seek to alleviate suffering. Editing aspects of aging does not absolve us of the need to confront mortality honestly and to support dignified dying when the time comes.

Cultural perspectives on aging vary widely, shaping how societies respond to the idea of slowing or editing it. In some traditions, elders are revered as sources of wisdom and continuity, and longevity is seen as a blessing to be shared. In others, aging may be more associated with decline, invisibility, or burden. Biotechnological interventions do not occur in a vacuum; they interact with these existing narratives, potentially reinforcing or challenging them. If extended healthspan becomes more common, it could amplify ageism if older people are expected to remain endlessly "productive," or it could foster a broader reimagining of life stages with room for multiple careers, reinvention, and extended learning. How we talk about aging scientifically will influence how we talk about it culturally, and vice versa.

Measuring success in editing aging itself requires more than counting extra years. Researchers and policymakers must track metrics like disability-free life expectancy, cognitive function, social engagement, and subjective well-being. A therapy that adds years of severe frailty and dependency would be a poor bargain compared with one that delays disease onset and preserves autonomy. People often say they want to "add life to years, not just years to life," and longevity science must take this seriously. Clinical trials for aging-targeted interventions are beginning to use composite endpoints that reflect multiple domains of health, rather than focusing on a single disease. This more holistic view aligns with the lived experience of aging, where mobility, cognition, mood, and social ties matter together.

In practical terms, the first widely adopted "aging therapies" may look less like elixirs of youth and more like repurposed medications that slightly shift risk curves. A drug originally developed for diabetes might be found to reduce the incidence of several age-related diseases when taken by older adults. A senolytic regimen could modestly improve physical function and reduce inflammatory markers in those with early frailty. These incremental gains, applied at population scale, could have large aggregate effects on health systems and quality of life. Over time, combinations of lifestyle, pharmacologic, and perhaps cellular interventions might form personalized aging-management plans, tailored to each person's risks, preferences, and values.

The prospect of editing aging also invites reflection on what we consider a "good" lifespan. Is there an ideal length of life, or is our goal to support health for as long as biological and ecological realities allow. How do we balance individual desires for longevity with responsibilities to future generations and the planet. These questions do not have simple answers, and they cannot be settled by scientists alone. They require dialogue among ethicists, faith communities, policymakers, and citizens across ages and cultures. Longevity science provides new tools and possibilities; society must decide how to wield them.

In the narrative of this book, editing aging itself sits at the intersection of many biotechnological themes. Genomics helps identify risk pathways, gene therapies and editing offer precise interventions, regenerative medicine attempts to restore tissue function, immunotherapies recalibrate defenses, and smart diagnostics track changes over time. Together, they form a toolkit that could reshape how we think about the later decades of life.

The challenge is to ensure that in our efforts to push back the boundaries of decline, we do not lose sight of what makes added years meaningful: relationships, purpose, creativity, and the freedom to live in ways we value. As we turn next to how biotech is reshaping care at the bedside, we will see how some of these aging-focused insights are already influencing everyday clinical practice, even as more ambitious interventions remain on the horizon.

Chapter .14

Biotech at the Bedside

Hospitals and clinics are being reshaped by advanced biotech tools and treatments.

For many people, the most vivid experience of biotechnology is not in a research article or news headline, but in a hospital room. It is the infusion pump that delivers a precisely calculated dose of a monoclonal antibody. It is the lab result that comes back with a genetic profile of a tumor. It is the handheld scanner that shows blood flow in an artery or the tablet that maps vital signs in real time. Over the last few decades, a quiet transformation has been unfolding at the bedside, where once-experimental tools have become part of daily clinical routine. This chapter is about that transformation: how biotech moves from bench to bedside, what it feels like for patients and clinicians, and how it changes the very texture of care. It is one thing to read about precision medicine and gene therapy in theory; it is another to watch how they show up in an ordinary ward on a Tuesday afternoon.

One of the most visible changes is how diagnoses are made. In the past, many conditions were identified using a combination of physical examination, basic lab tests, and imaging that provided relatively coarse information. Today, bedside decisions increasingly draw on molecular diagnostics that slice disease into finer and finer categories. A person arriving with a suspicious lump may not just hear "you have breast cancer," but "you have a tumor that over-expresses this receptor, carries these mutations, and is likely to respond to that targeted agent." A patient with an infection may have the responsible microbe identified not only by culture, but by rapid genetic tests that also reveal which antibiotics it will resist. These layers of detail do not replace clinical judgment, but they give it a sharper edge, helping clinicians choose treatments that fit the specific biology in front of them.

This molecular detail filters through the life of the hospital in subtle ways. Pathology labs increasingly rely on panels of biomarkers, gene expression signatures, and sequencing results alongside slides under a microscope. Infectious disease teams consult resistance profiles generated by machines that read bacterial DNA as easily as older instruments read glucose. Transplant teams match donors and recipients using broader sets of immune markers, trying to reduce rejection and improve graft survival. In many cases, the samples are small—tiny tubes of blood, tissue, or swabs—but the information extracted is enormous. The bedside conversation might still be simple—"this antibiotic should work better for you"—yet behind it lies a web of biotechnology humming quietly in the background.

Monoclonal antibodies are another example of biotech settling into everyday practice. These engineered proteins are designed to bind specific targets in the body, from cancer cells to inflammatory molecules. They are now prescribed for cancers, autoimmune diseases, migraines, and more, often administered through infusions in clinics or hospitals. For patients, the experience may look straightforward: sit in a reclining chair, have an IV placed, and watch a bag slowly empty. But that clear liquid carries years of design, testing, and manufacturing optimization. Nurses monitor for infusion reactions, pharmacists calculate doses based on body weight or biomarker levels, and clinicians adjust schedules depending on how the disease responds. What was once cutting-edge is now a routine part of many infusion suites, where rows of chairs and beeping pumps form the front line of biotech at the bedside.

Cellular therapies, such as CAR-T cells and certain stem cell transplants, bring an even more direct presence of biotechnology into the ward. Preparing a patient for these treatments can involve detailed planning, preconditioning chemotherapy, and coordination with specialized labs that handle the cells. When the engineered cells finally arrive—often in a small bag thawed from frozen storage—the moment can feel deceptively ordinary. The infusion may take only minutes, looking much like a blood transfusion. Yet everyone in the room understands that this is different: living cells carrying customized genetic instructions are entering the body, with the potential to expand, persist, and fundamentally reshape disease. Afterward, clinicians monitor closely for side effects, such as immune storms or neurological changes, ready to intervene quickly. The boundary between therapy and the patient's own biology becomes blurred; the treatment is no longer just something given but something that can continue to act from within.

Regenerative medicine also has a bedside face. In orthopedic wards, cartilage repair procedures may use scaffolds seeded with cells or biologic injectables that aim to support tissue healing rather than simply replacing joints with prosthetics. Burn units may apply bioengineered skin substitutes that combine cells and biomaterials, reducing scarring and infection. In cardiac care, patients might be enrolled in trials where cells or growth factors are delivered to damaged hearts in hopes of enhancing recovery. Each of these interventions comes wrapped in ordinary hospital routines—consent forms, anesthesia, post-op checks—but they carry a different intention: not just patching, but persuading the body to rebuild. Outcomes are still mixed in many areas, and expectations must be managed carefully. Yet even experimental procedures change the culture of the bedside, teaching clinicians and patients to think in terms of repair and regeneration rather than only replacement.

Biotech at the bedside is not limited to drugs and cells; it includes the devices that monitor and support patients moment to moment. Ventilators, dialysis machines, and extracorporeal membrane oxygenation circuits (ECMO) have all grown more sophisticated, guided by sensors and algorithms that adjust flows and pressures continuously. Bedside ultrasound, once the domain of specialists, is spreading to general wards and emergency departments through compact, portable units that fit in a pocket. Nurses and physicians can quickly scan the heart, lungs, or abdomen, gaining real-time insight that previously required sending patients to distant imaging suites. These devices are not purely "biotech" in the narrow sense, but they embody the fusion of biology, engineering, and informatics that characterizes modern care. They make the bedside feel less like a static location and more like an adaptable, miniaturized diagnostic lab.

Electronic health records and decision-support systems are another, less visible, dimension of biotech in clinical settings. On rounds, clinicians move from bed to bed armed with tablets or workstations that display lab trends, imaging, and risk scores generated by algorithms. When they order medications, the system checks for dangerous interactions, kidney function, and genetic variants that might affect dosing. Alerts pop up when vital signs drift into concerning patterns or when lab results suggest sepsis or heart injury. Done well, this digital layer supports safer, more consistent care, catching errors before they reach patients. Done poorly, it can overwhelm clinicians with pop-ups and clicks, pulling attention away from the person in the bed toward the screen. Balancing the benefits of digital biotech with the need for human presence is an ongoing challenge that plays out every day in hospitals around the world.

Biotech innovations also reshape the physical flow of patients through the healthcare system. Rapid molecular tests in emergency departments can quickly distinguish between viral and bacterial infections, reducing unnecessary antibiotic use and helping decide who needs admission and who can go home. Point-of-care troponin assays and imaging tools help triage chest pain, guiding some patients straight to the catheterization lab while reassuring others. In oncology clinics, the timing of infusions can be aligned with biomarker results, reducing wasted trips and delays. Behind the scenes, hospital pharmacies adopt new biomanufacturing methods to prepare sterile, individualized doses of advanced therapies. The path from arrival to discharge becomes less linear and more tailored, guided by technologies that reveal more about each patient's risks and needs.

For clinicians, working in a biotech-rich environment changes the skills and knowledge they need. Training increasingly includes not only anatomy, physiology, and pharmacology, but also familiarity with genomic reports, cell therapy protocols, and device interfaces. Trainees learn how to interpret variant classifications, weigh the implications of a molecular test, and counsel patients about the uncertain meaning of some findings. They also learn to collaborate with specialized teams: genetic counselors, molecular pathologists, pharmacists, and data scientists who bring expertise in particular technologies. The bedside becomes a shared space where multiple disciplines converge, each contributing a piece of the puzzle. Communication and humility are essential, because no single person can master all the technologies now in play.

From the patient's perspective, biotech at the bedside can be both reassuring and overwhelming. On one hand, it can inspire confidence to know that care is guided by refined tests and modern tools, that therapies are designed specifically for the type of disease they have, and that monitoring is continuous and precise. On the other hand, the array of machines, drips, and acronyms can feel alien and intimidating. Many people do not want a deep lecture on molecular pathways when they are tired and afraid; they want to understand, in plain language, what is happening to them and why. The task of clinicians, therefore, is not only to deploy biotech wisely but to translate its implications into stories and choices that patients can grasp. Even the most advanced therapy must ultimately be explained in terms of what it means for pain, mobility, energy, and time with loved ones.

Equity issues are especially stark at the bedside, where differences in access to biotech become visible in who gets which tests and treatments. In some hospitals, patients can receive comprehensive genomic profiling, cutting-edge cell therapies, and advanced biologics as part of routine care. In others, basic lab tests and older drugs may be the only options, constrained by resources, insurance coverage, or geography. Even within the same institution, disparities can arise based on language, insurance status, or implicit biases. A person who speaks the dominant language fluently and advocates assertively for themselves may be more likely to be offered experimental therapies than someone who is quieter or faces systemic discrimination. Addressing these gaps requires more than technology; it demands conscious policies, outreach, and training to ensure that biotech advances do not deepen existing injustices.

Safety and ethics remain central as biotech tools become more embedded in bedside practice. Every new therapy—whether a gene-modifying infusion, a potent biologic, or an AI-driven monitoring system—carries unknowns when first introduced. Hospitals develop protocols, consent forms, and oversight committees to manage these uncertainties, but the real testing ground is always the lived experience of patients and staff. When side effects occur, or when algorithms misfire, trust can be shaken. Transparent reporting, rapid learning, and honest communication about risks and benefits are essential to maintaining that trust. The bedside is where the promises of biotech are judged not by theoretical potential but by outcomes, complications, and the ways in which people feel heard and respected.

There is also the question of how much technology is too much. Some clinicians worry about "monitoring fatigue," where constant streams of data lead to over-testing, over-treating, and increased anxiety without necessarily improving outcomes. For example, detecting every minor abnormality on a scan or every transient blip in a heart rhythm might lead to cascades of investigations and interventions that carry their own risks. Biotech at the bedside must therefore be paired with wise restraint, recognizing when not to act as much as when to act. This kind of restraint grows out of experience, evidence, and conversations with patients about what they value. More tools do not automatically mean more interventions; sometimes they enable more confident decisions to watch and wait.

Teaching hospitals and clinical trials are often the first places where new biotechnologies touch patients, serving as bridges between research and routine care. Here, the bedside becomes a site of experimentation, with protocols comparing standard treatments to innovative ones under controlled conditions. Patients who enroll in these trials may receive access to therapies not yet widely available, but they also accept added uncertainty and frequent monitoring. Ethics committees, regulatory bodies, and patient advocates work to ensure that this research is conducted fairly, with informed consent and appropriate safeguards. The knowledge gained flows outward, shaping guidelines and practices that will eventually reach many more hospitals and clinics. In this way, the bedside is not only a destination for biotech; it is also a source of evidence that feeds back into the wider scientific ecosystem.

In the broader arc of this book, biotech at the bedside represents the point where abstract innovations become tangible experiences. Gene editing, regenerative medicine, immunotherapies, organs-on-chips, synthetic biology, and AI all converge here, translated into protocols, devices, and conversations. A single hospital room might contain a person receiving a monoclonal antibody designed through structural biology, monitored by wearables feeding data into AI algorithms, with treatment decisions informed by genomic sequencing and modeled on organ-on-chip studies. Yet none of this will matter if the person in that bed feels alone, confused, or dismissed. The ultimate test of biotech is not only whether it works in biological terms, but whether it enhances the human experience of illness and healing. As we move in the next chapter to at-home biotech, we will see how these tools continue their journey beyond hospital walls, following people into the spaces where most of life —and most of health—actually happens.

Chapter .15

At-Home Biotech

Direct-to-consumer tests and digital tools are bringing biotech capabilities into the home.

For most people, "biotechnology" used to mean buildings far away: research labs with white coats and whirring machines, or hospitals full of complex equipment. Today, a growing share of biotech has moved into kitchens, bathrooms, and living rooms. A saliva kit on the dining table, a blood pressure cuff on the shelf, a phone app that interprets lab results—these have become part of everyday life for many. At-home biotech blurs the distinction between patient and consumer, clinic and couch. It gives individuals tools to measure, explore, and sometimes even intervene in their own biology without waiting for a doctor's order. This shift offers new opportunities for empowerment and prevention, but it also brings new risks of confusion, anxiety, and inequity.

Direct-to-consumer genetic tests are among the most recognizable faces of at-home biotech. For the price of a nice dinner out, people can spit into a tube, mail it off, and receive reports about ancestry, certain traits, and limited health information. Some companies focus on where a person's ancestors may have lived centuries ago; others highlight variants associated with metabolism, drug response, or disease risk. For many users, the experience is partly entertainment and partly self-exploration. They may discover unexpected branches in their family tree or learn why cilantro tastes like soap. At the same time, the presence of health-related findings can turn a casual curiosity into a weighty matter. A single line in a report hinting at elevated risk for a disease can change how someone feels about their future, even when the actual increase in risk is modest.

The appeal of at-home genetic tests lies in their simplicity and immediacy. No appointment is needed, no waiting room, no need to convince a clinician that a test is warranted. Results are delivered via colorful dashboards and interactive graphs rather than dense lab printouts. Yet the very qualities that make them accessible also make them easy to misunderstand. Risk percentages may be interpreted as destiny, and uncertainty is often hard to convey in a cheerful app interface. People may not realize that many variants reported are only weakly associated with outcomes, or that environment and behavior can overwhelm small genetic nudges. Without guidance, some users may make drastic decisions or experience unnecessary worry based on information that clinicians would interpret quite differently.

In response to these challenges, a parallel ecosystem has emerged around at-home testing: online genetic counseling services, physician-ordered confirmatory tests, and educational resources that help put results in context. Some companies now allow or require users to connect with health professionals before seeing certain high-stakes findings, such as variants strongly linked to cancer risk. Others clearly separate ancestry and fun trait reports from medically significant information, encouraging users not to overinterpret the latter without professional input. Even so, the line between consumer curiosity and medical testing remains fuzzy. At-home biotech has effectively created a new front door to health information, one that opens before a person ever steps into a clinic.

Genetics is only one part of the at-home biotech landscape. Simple finger-prick kits now allow people to measure cholesterol, vitamin levels, hormone concentrations, and inflammatory markers from home, sending samples to certified labs and viewing results online. Rapid antigen tests for infections can be done on a kitchen counter, with results in minutes. Some companies bundle multiple biomarkers into "wellness panels" that promise insights into stress, metabolism, or immune status. The idea is to give individuals a more continuous picture of their internal state, rather than relying solely on annual checkups. For people who live far from clinics, or who face barriers to accessing traditional care, these tools can fill important gaps. They can also provide practical feedback for those making lifestyle changes or adjusting medications in collaboration with their clinicians.

Yet, like genetic tests, at-home lab kits come with interpretive challenges. A single elevated value may not mean much without context, and normal ranges are not absolute fences between health and disease. A slightly abnormal result could be a temporary blip, a lab variation, or the first hint of a significant problem. Distinguishing among these possibilities often requires medical training, knowledge of the person's history, and sometimes repeat testing. When results arrive directly in an inbox without explanation, people may either panic or ignore them entirely. The most helpful at-home systems therefore include clear, plain-language explanations, trend tracking, and easy pathways to consult clinicians. They treat data as the beginning of a conversation, not the end of it.

Biotech in the home also includes devices that monitor physiology in real time, extending the themes of wearables into more specialized tools. Portable blood pressure cuffs, home spirometers for lung function, and pulse oximeters for oxygen levels are now widely available and relatively affordable. People with chronic conditions such as hypertension, asthma, or heart failure can track their status daily, adjusting medications or behaviors based on agreed-upon plans with their care teams. This shifts some responsibility and power from the clinic to the household, allowing earlier detection of flares and reducing unnecessary visits. It also relies on trust: trust that people will use the devices correctly, that they will not be blamed for "bad numbers," and that clinicians will take their home data seriously. When that trust is present, at-home monitoring can make care feel more collaborative and less episodic.

Smartphone cameras and microphones have become surprisingly capable diagnostic tools. Apps can analyze photos of skin lesions for concerning features, record breathing to assess wheeze or snoring, and even measure heart rate and respiratory rate from subtle color changes in the face. While these tools are not replacements for in-person evaluation, they can act as preliminary screens that help people decide when to seek care and what to mention. A parent might use an app to track a child's rash over several days, capturing images that help a pediatrician distinguish allergies from infection. An older adult with chronic lung disease might send recordings of their cough to a clinician, who can spot changes early. In this sense, at-home biotech turns everyday devices into front-line observers of health, capturing data that would otherwise be lost.

The concept of "smart homes" is beginning to intersect with biotech, blurring the boundary between health monitoring and daily living. Sensors embedded in floors, mattresses, and appliances can track movement, sleep patterns, and even gait stability, sometimes without the person needing to wear or activate anything. For older adults or those with mobility challenges, such systems can detect falls, changes in activity that might signal illness, or wandering behavior in dementia. Alerts can be sent to caregivers or emergency services, providing a safety net that extends beyond traditional call buttons. At their best, these technologies support independence and peace of mind, allowing people to stay in their homes longer. At their worst, they can feel intrusive or paternalistic, especially if implemented without clear consent and control.

At-home biotech is not confined to passive measurement; it increasingly includes active interventions. Telemedicine platforms, combined with home diagnostics, allow clinicians to prescribe treatments remotely, adjust doses based on real-time data, and oversee programs like physical therapy or cardiac rehabilitation through video and sensor feedback. Some companies ship kits that include not only test materials but also starter medications or devices, all coordinated via app. In reproductive health, at-home ovulation tests, fertility hormone tracking, and sperm analysis allow couples to gather detailed information without visiting a clinic. In mental health, digital therapeutics—software-based treatments for conditions like insomnia or anxiety—deliver structured behavioral programs validated in clinical trials, sometimes prescribed like a medication but "taken" on a phone.

The rise of at-home biotech has also fueled a movement of do-it-yourself biology, or "DIY bio," where enthusiasts explore experiments outside traditional institutions. Community labs offer shared space and equipment for hobbyists, students, and citizen scientists to learn molecular biology, grow microbes, or tinker with genetic constructs under supervision. Some individuals experiment with self-tracking and self-experimentation, adjusting diets, supplements, or routines and monitoring biomarkers to see what happens. At its best, this culture fosters curiosity, democratizes scientific literacy, and can even contribute to innovation. At its worst, unsupervised or poorly informed experimentation risks harm, especially when it strays into areas like unapproved gene therapies or untested injections. Responsible DIY communities emphasize safety, ethics, and respect for legal boundaries, but the broader environment remains uneven.

Equity and access issues are woven deeply into the story of at-home biotech. The ability to order mail-in tests, use apps, and interpret results assumes stable housing, reliable mail service, and access to smartphones or computers. It assumes literacy in at least one major language and enough free time and mental bandwidth to learn new interfaces. People who work multiple jobs, lack broadband, or face caregiving burdens may find even "simple" at-home tools difficult to use. If health systems start to expect patients to monitor and manage more from home without providing support, there is a risk that those already under strain will be left further behind. Addressing this requires designing tools with diverse users in mind, offering alternative pathways, and integrating at-home biotech into community clinics and outreach programs rather than only marketing directly to individuals.

Privacy concerns are especially salient when biotech moves into the home. Data collected from tests, apps, and devices may be stored by companies that are not bound by the same confidentiality rules as traditional healthcare providers. Information about genetics, fertility, mental health, or substance use could, in theory, be shared with advertisers, employers, or insurers if protections are weak. Even within households, at-home tests can raise sensitive questions: who sees the results, who controls the accounts, and how are family members' data respected. Clear consent processes, robust data protection, and options to delete or export information are essential to earn and keep trust. People should not have to trade privacy for access to useful tools.

At-home biotech is also changing how clinicians work. When patients arrive at appointments with printouts, spreadsheets, or app dashboards full of data, clinicians must decide what to focus on and how to incorporate it into their assessments. Some data will be highly relevant; other elements may be misleading or redundant. Clinicians may need to say, "This particular test is not validated in your situation," or "Let's not worry about that marker; here's what matters most." Building this kind of interpretive capacity into everyday practice takes time and training. It can also be emotionally delicate, as people may feel attached to the effort they put into gathering data. Respectful dialogue that acknowledges patients' initiative while gently correcting misunderstandings can strengthen relationships rather than straining them.

Education is a crucial pillar supporting safe and effective use of at-home biotech. People do not need PhDs to benefit from these tools, but they do need a basic grasp of concepts like risk, variability, and false positives. Simple explanations—about why a single abnormal result is not a verdict, why trends over time matter, and why some findings require confirmation—can prevent unnecessary distress. Educational materials embedded within apps and test kits, as well as public health campaigns that address common misconceptions, can help. Schools and community organizations can also play a role, integrating basic health literacy and data literacy into curricula. The more people understand about how these tools work and what their limits are, the more likely they are to use them wisely.

On a more hopeful note, at-home biotech has the potential to strengthen the connection between daily life and long-term health in tangible ways. Seeing blood pressure numbers improve after a change in diet, or sleep patterns stabilize after adjusting routines, can make abstract advice feel real. For people who have felt dismissed or disempowered in traditional medical settings, gaining access to their own data can be validating. It can provide evidence to support their descriptions of symptoms and responses to treatment. When linked with supportive clinicians, at-home tools can transform the patient role from passive recipient to active participant, without expecting people to become their own doctors.

At the same time, there is a risk that constant self-measurement can tip into self-surveillance, where every fluctuation feels like a flaw to be corrected. Some people find that tracking weight, sleep, or food intake intensively worsens anxiety or obsessive tendencies. Others may feel judged by apps that set "ideal" targets without understanding their lived realities. Designing at-home biotech with mental health in mind—offering flexible goals, emphasizing self-compassion, and providing options to step back from tracking when needed—is as important as calibrating its sensors. Health is not only about numbers; it is also about how people feel about themselves while they pursue change.

In the broader arc of biotechnology, at-home tools represent a decentralization of power and information. Where once the only route to advanced testing or monitoring was through large institutions, individuals now have increasing ability to initiate measurements and store records themselves. This shift can support more personalized, continuous care, especially when there are strong bridges between home and clinic. It also means that decisions about which tools to trust, which companies to engage with, and how to interpret data are moving closer to the front door. Building a culture that supports wise use of at-home biotech—

through education, regulation, and equitable design—will shape whether this revolution enhances health for many or mainly benefits a privileged few.

As we move from this chapter into the ethics of engineered life, it is worth pausing on a simple image: a person sitting at a kitchen table, opening a small box that contains a test kit, a device, or a new app. In that ordinary moment, decades of scientific work, policy, and design coalesce into a choice: to swab, to spit, to prick, to track—or to set the box aside. At-home biotech makes those choices more frequent and more consequential. The question is not just what the tools can do, but how we as individuals and societies decide to invite them into our homes, our relationships, and our sense of who we are.

Author Reflection – At-Home Biotech

Writing about at-home biotech, I kept picturing small, quiet moments: a parent carefully reading the instructions on a test strip, an elder scrolling through heart-rate graphs on a tablet, a teenager wondering what a genetic result really means. None of these scenes involve dramatic machines or operating rooms, yet they are where biotechnology meets daily life most intimately. I am struck by how much trust is implied in these moments—trust in companies we may never meet, trust in our own ability to interpret data, and trust that someone will help us when results are confusing or scary. At-home tools can feel empowering, but they can also feel lonely if they are not connected to supportive communities and clinicians. My hope is that as these technologies spread, we remember that sending kits and apps into people's homes is not enough; we must also send understanding, empathy, and clear pathways to human help.

Inspirational Quotes

A test on the kitchen table is more than a gadget; it is an invitation to know ourselves more deeply and to decide what we will do with that knowledge.

Chapter .16

Ethics in the Age of Engineered Life

Society must decide where to draw the line between treating disease, enhancing humans, and designing life.

Ethics in biotechnology often begins not with abstract principles, but with very concrete questions: who gets offered a new therapy, who bears the risks, and who decides when enough is enough. Every infusion of a gene therapy, every embryo tested in an IVF clinic, and every engineered cell put into a patient's body carries choices that reach beyond the individuals involved. They touch on beliefs about fairness, normality, and what makes a life "worth" living. In the age of engineered life, these choices are no longer just about whether to accept or refuse treatment, but about which possibilities we are willing to create in the first place. Each new technology we develop invites us, quietly or loudly, to redraw the line between what we consider natural and what we are willing to design. Those lines are rarely fixed, and they are never purely scientific.

One of the first ethical distinctions people make is between treating disease and enhancing traits. Treating disease usually means restoring function that has been lost or impaired, aligning a body more closely with what we consider typical. Enhancing traits, by contrast, suggests going beyond the usual range, adding capabilities or features that confer advantage. On paper, this seems like a clear division, but in practice the boundary blurs. Correcting a gene that causes severe anemia looks like treatment, yet what about boosting a normal person's red blood cell capacity for athletic performance. Helping a child hear through a cochlear implant addresses disability, but some in Deaf communities see deafness as a cultural identity, not a defect to be fixed. Ethics in engineered life must grapple with these ambiguities, recognizing that "treatment" and "enhancement" are shaped by culture, history, and power, not just by biology.

The question of normality runs through many debates about biotechnology. When we talk about correcting abnormalities, we imply that there is a standard body or mind to which people should conform. That standard often reflects the experiences and preferences of those in positions of authority, leaving less room for forms of difference that are inconvenient, poorly understood, or stigmatized. Engineering life can either reinforce narrow ideals or expand our appreciation for diversity, depending on how it is used. If genetic screening and editing are focused only on eliminating certain conditions, we risk sending the message that those lives are less valuable. On the other hand, if we use technology to reduce suffering while also honoring the dignity of those who live with difference, we can resist that harmful implication. Ethics in biotech is not just about what we can change, but about what we choose to celebrate and accommodate rather than erase.

Genetic screening in reproduction brings these questions into particularly sharp relief. Prospective parents can now test embryos for certain chromosomal abnormalities, monogenic diseases, and, increasingly, polygenic risk profiles linked to complex traits. They may face decisions about which embryos to implant, which pregnancies to continue, and which risks they are willing to accept. For some families, avoiding a condition that has caused profound pain is an act of love and responsibility. For others, the very act of selection feels deeply troubling, as if they are ranking potential lives by desirability. On a societal level, widespread use of reproductive technologies can shape which conditions become rarer and which remain common, subtly engineering the future population. This raises fears of new forms of eugenics, driven not by state coercion but by market forces, social pressure, and biased ideas about what counts as a "good" life.

Somatic gene editing, which affects only the treated individual, and germline editing, which alters future generations, present different ethical landscapes. Somatic interventions focus on people who are already alive and can, in principle, consent to risks and benefits. Germline editing, by contrast, changes the genetic inheritance of descendants who cannot consent and who may experience unintended consequences. Many scientific and ethical bodies argue that germline editing for clinical use should remain off-limits, at least for now, given the uncertainties and the potential for misuse. They call for strong international norms and oversight to prevent rushed experiments that could have lasting harms. The challenge is that technical capabilities often advance faster than global agreements, and individual actors can act unilaterally. Ethics in the age of engineered life must therefore be proactive, not only reacting to controversies after the fact but setting guardrails before temptations become too strong.

Consent becomes more complicated when interventions involve communities, not just individuals. For example, releasing genetically modified mosquitoes to reduce disease transmission affects entire regions, including people who may never have heard of the technology. Similarly, using shared health and genomic data to build AI models or identify new drug targets draws on the contributions of many, each with their own expectations. Meaningful consent in such contexts cannot be reduced to a single form or click-through agreement. It requires ongoing dialogue, community engagement, and mechanisms for people to voice concerns and withdraw participation where possible. At a deeper level, it demands recognizing that some groups—especially those historically marginalized—may view research and medical institutions with understandable mistrust, shaped by past abuses. Ethical biotech must take that history seriously, not just as background, but as something to be actively repaired.

Justice is a central concern when powerful technologies risk being distributed unevenly. Biotech innovations are often expensive when first introduced, available primarily in advanced centers and wealthy health systems. This pattern is familiar from other areas of medicine, but it becomes more troubling as interventions move closer to altering the basic conditions of health and lifespan. If gene therapies, regenerative treatments, or aging-targeted drugs are available only to those who can pay high prices, we risk entrenching biological privilege on top of existing economic and social privilege. Even within countries with public health systems, disparities can arise based on geography, advocacy, and subtle forms of bias. Ethical reflection cannot stop at "is this safe and effective"; it must ask "who is left out, and what are we doing to include them."

Data ethics has become inseparable from biotechnology ethics, because so many modern tools rely on large datasets of genomes, health records, and sensor readings. Questions of privacy, ownership, and benefit-sharing are not mere technicalities; they touch on people's sense of autonomy and trust. When someone contributes their DNA to a research project, who gets to decide how it is used in future studies. Should they or their community share in profits if a lucrative therapy is built on their data. How do we protect individuals from re-identification, discrimination, or surveillance based on biological information. These questions do not have easy answers, but avoiding them is itself an ethical choice —one that usually benefits those already in control of the data. Responsible biotech asks not only "Can we analyze this," but also "Should we, under what conditions, and with what return to those who contributed."

Cultural and religious perspectives shape ethical views on engineered life in powerful ways. Concepts of what is sacred, what is natural, and what constitutes harm vary widely across traditions. For some, manipulating embryos or mixing human and animal cells crosses moral boundaries that feel inviolable. For others, healing through any available means is a fulfillment of spiritual duty, and drawing strict lines between natural and artificial is less meaningful. Ethical frameworks that ignore these plural perspectives risk imposing a narrow worldview through technology. At the same time, simply saying "everyone has their own opinion" is not enough when policies must be made and practices regulated. The task is to build deliberative spaces—citizen assemblies, interfaith dialogues, participatory councils—where diverse voices can be heard and where trade-offs are openly discussed.

The possibility of human enhancement raises especially charged questions about fairness and identity. If safe methods emerged to boost cognitive performance, improve physical endurance, or alter emotional resilience, who would use them and why. Would they be limited to treating clearly defined impairments, or would they become tools for competition in school, work, and sports. Historical experience suggests that whenever performance-enhancing technologies appear, pressures arise to use them simply to keep up. In such a world, saying "no" can feel less like a free choice and more like self-sabotage. Ethics in enhancement is therefore not just about individual risk–benefit calculations; it is about the social contexts that make some choices feel compulsory. It invites us to ask what kinds of excellence we value and whether we can build societies where dignity does not depend on constantly optimized performance.

The line between human and non-human life also becomes blurred in the age of bioengineering. Chimeric organisms—those containing cells from more than one species—can be powerful research tools, helping us model diseases or grow human-compatible organs in animals. At the same time, they raise questions about moral status, especially when human neural tissues are involved. Similarly, organoids and brain-like structures grown in the lab have prompted philosophical debate about whether, at some level of complexity, they might have experiences we should care about. Most current models are far from any plausible threshold of consciousness, but ethics asks us to think ahead: if and when systems approach that threshold, how will we recognize it, and what obligations will we have. Treating all such concerns as science fiction would be a mistake; thoughtful boundaries and monitoring mechanisms can be designed now, before lines are accidentally crossed.

Regulation is one of the main tools societies use to express ethical priorities in biotechnology, but its design is tricky. Too little regulation can invite reckless experimentation, exploitation, and erosion of trust; too much can stifle beneficial innovation and drive risky work into unregulated corners. Different countries adopt different balances, reflecting their own histories and political cultures. Some emphasize precaution, demanding strong evidence of safety and social value before approving new technologies. Others lean toward permissiveness, relying on market forces and professional norms to self-correct. Because biotech crosses borders easily—through data, reagents, and know-how—purely national approaches have limits. International guidelines, transparent reporting, and cross-border collaborations can help ensure that no one jurisdiction becomes a haven for practices widely considered unacceptable.

Public communication plays a critical ethical role in the age of engineered life. How technologies are described to the public influences expectations, fears, and support for research. Hype and overselling can create unrealistic hopes that leave patients feeling misled and betrayed when results fall short. Alarmist narratives can provoke panic or resistance that is out of proportion to actual risks. Ethical communication aims for honesty about uncertainty, avoids promises of miracles, and respects the intelligence of the audience. It acknowledges both the potential and the limitations of biotechnology, and it is upfront about who funded the work and who stands to gain. Informed publics are better able to participate in decisions about what research to support, what regulations to endorse, and when to push back.

Another dimension of ethics concerns how we relate to non-medical uses of biotechnology, such as cosmetic gene editing or designer pets. As techniques become more accessible, people may be tempted to use them for vanity or novelty rather than health. A company might offer to adjust minor traits in embryos to match trends or aesthetics, while others might propose genetically modified animals as status symbols. These uses may seem trivial compared with life-saving therapies, yet they shape cultural norms around what is acceptable to modify. If we normalize editing for superficial reasons, it may become harder to draw lines when more consequential changes are proposed. Ethics here is less about individual harm and more about what kind of relationship to life we want to cultivate: one of stewardship and respect, or one of endless customization.

Responsibility in biotechnology is often distributed across many actors, making accountability complex. A problematic outcome from a gene therapy trial might be traced back to decisions by scientists, regulators, companies, clinicians, and investors. Likewise, the exclusion of certain groups from access to a technology might reflect biases in funding, clinical trial design, insurance coverage, and public policy. Ethical analyses that focus only on individual bad actors miss these systemic dimensions. A more robust approach asks how incentives, structures, and narratives combine to produce patterns of harm or neglect. It pushes for changes at multiple levels: not just better training for individual practitioners, but also reforms in how research is funded, how success is measured, and how benefits are shared.

Education, both for professionals and the public, is a key ethical lever. Scientists and clinicians need training not only in technical skills but also in ethical reasoning, cultural humility, and communication. Bioethics should not be a one-time course, but an ongoing conversation woven into research meetings, clinical rounds, and regulatory hearings. Likewise, members of the public benefit from accessible education about genetics, risk, and the basics of clinical research. A population that understands how studies are designed, what consent means, and how to interpret claims about therapies is less vulnerable to exploitation by quack treatments or misleading marketing. Education is not about dictating what people should think, but about equipping them with tools to think clearly and independently about complex choices.

Finally, ethics in the age of engineered life reminds us that technology alone cannot tell us what a good life is. Biotech may help us live longer, suffer less from disease, or express our identities more fully, but it cannot answer questions about purpose, belonging, and meaning. Those questions arise in families, communities, philosophies, and spiritual traditions. Ethical reflection invites us to keep those conversations alive even as technical possibilities expand. It asks us to pause before each new capability and consider not just whether we can implement it safely, but how it fits into the stories we tell about who we are and who we hope to be. When we do that, engineering life becomes less about control and more about care—care for bodies, for communities, and for the fragile world that sustains us.

In the flow of this book, ethics is not a separate chapter bolted onto the end of scientific discussion; it is a thread that runs through every topic. Still, pausing to focus on it explicitly matters, because it frames how we approach all that comes next. As we turn to questions of access, equity, and the global biotech divide, we will see how ethical aspirations meet real-world constraints. The best principles in the world mean little if they are not translated into who receives treatment, who gets left waiting, and how we respond to the widening gaps that advanced medicine can create. Ethics, in that sense, is not just about what we believe, but about what we are willing to build and share.

Chapter .17

Access, Equity, and the Global Biotech Divide

Biotech advances risk widening global inequality unless access gaps are deliberately addressed.

Whenever a new breakthrough therapy is announced, the first question many people ask is, "Does it work." For billions of others, a more pressing question follows quickly: "Will it ever be available where I live, and if so, when." The distance between those two questions is the space where the global biotech divide lives. Advanced diagnostics, targeted drugs, and gene therapies are often born in well-funded labs and rolled out first in wealthy health systems. Meanwhile, clinics with intermittent electricity, limited staff, and shortages of basic medicines struggle to provide even routine care. Without deliberate effort, each new biotech success risks layering another level of advantage onto those who already have the most, while leaving others further behind. The challenge is not only scientific; it is deeply political, economic, and moral.

The divide shows up starkly in access to essential medicines that are no longer new at all. Vaccines, insulin, cancer drugs, and treatments for HIV have transformed health outcomes in many countries, yet remain scarce, unaffordable, or inconsistently available in others. Patents, pricing strategies, fragile supply chains, and weak health systems all play a role. A life-saving biologic may exist on the shelf of a hospital in one city while being effectively nonexistent in a rural clinic a few hundred kilometers away. Even within the same country, people in wealthy neighborhoods may receive state-of-the-art therapies while those in informal settlements struggle to see a clinician at all. Biotech does not create these inequities, but it can amplify them when high-cost, complex interventions are layered on top of already uneven foundations.

The infrastructure required to deploy advanced biotechnologies is itself unevenly distributed. Gene therapies, stem cell treatments, and complex biologics often need cold chains, specialized lab facilities, and highly trained teams to administer and monitor them safely. Many regions of the world lack reliable electricity, let alone dedicated cell-processing suites or high-throughput sequencers. Even when equipment is donated, maintenance, reagents, and staff training can be ongoing bottlenecks. As a result, global health organizations must weigh whether to invest limited resources in cutting-edge therapies for a few or in basic services—vaccination, safe childbirth, clean water—that benefit many. These are not purely technical decisions; they reflect values about whose lives are prioritized and how justice is defined in practice.

Cost is a powerful gatekeeper in the biotech era. New gene therapies and specialized cell treatments often launch with price tags in the hundreds of thousands or even millions of dollars per patient. Companies argue that these prices reflect years of research and the potential for long-term savings if conditions are cured rather than managed. Critics respond that such costs are simply incompatible with universal access, even in high-income countries. In low- and middle-income settings, they are beyond imagination. Tiered pricing, generics, biosimilars, and pooled purchasing can help, but they cannot fully bridge a gap when the starting point is so vast. Unless pricing and intellectual property models evolve, many of the most transformative biotechnologies will remain boutique solutions for a small, privileged subset of humanity.

Clinical trials, which determine how safe and effective new biotechnologies are, often mirror and reinforce global inequities. Many trials are concentrated in regions with existing research infrastructure and regulatory familiarity, often in North America, Europe, and parts of Asia. Populations from other regions may be underrepresented, meaning that results do not fully reflect genetic, environmental, and cultural diversity. When trials do occur in lower-resource settings, additional ethical questions arise. Participants may have limited access to standard care, raising concerns about undue inducement or exploitation. After a trial ends, the therapy may never become available locally, even if it proves successful. In such cases, communities bear the risks of research without sharing proportionately in its benefits, deepening mistrust and resentment.

The biotech divide is not only about geography; it is also about race, class, gender, and other axes of discrimination within countries. In many health systems, marginalized groups face barriers to advanced diagnostics and treatments even when those interventions exist nearby. Language differences, implicit bias, lack of insurance, and historical mistreatment can all limit access. For example, precision oncology trials may under-enroll patients from minority communities, leading to less robust data on how targeted drugs work for them. Meanwhile, algorithms used to allocate resources or predict risk can embed biases present in the data they were trained on, compounding disparities under a veil of objectivity. Addressing the global biotech divide therefore requires attention to internal inequities, not just differences between countries.

Digital technologies, including AI and telemedicine, offer both hope and hazard. On one hand, they can extend specialist expertise into remote clinics, support decision-making in under-resourced settings, and help manage chronic diseases with fewer in-person visits. On the other hand, they rely on electricity, internet connectivity, and devices that are still far from universally available. When AI models are trained on data from privileged populations, they may perform poorly in settings with different disease profiles and resource constraints. Telehealth platforms designed for people with high-end smartphones and unlimited data plans may be unusable for those sharing a single device or living in areas with patchy coverage. The digital divide and the biotech divide overlap, reinforcing each other in ways that must be consciously countered.

Local capacity building is widely recognized as a key strategy for narrowing the gap. Rather than relying solely on imported products and expertise, countries can invest in training scientists, clinicians, and regulators, as well as in local manufacturing of vaccines, diagnostics, and biologics. Technology transfer agreements, regional research networks, and south–south collaborations can accelerate this process. When local teams help design studies, prioritize health problems, and adapt technologies to their own contexts, solutions become more sustainable and culturally appropriate. Capacity building is not charity; it is a partnership that recognizes the knowledge and agency already present in communities. It also helps prevent situations where a few global hubs dictate which diseases are studied and which are neglected.

Intellectual property systems play a pivotal role in shaping who has access to biotech and when. Patents are intended to reward innovation by granting temporary monopolies, but when applied rigidly to life-saving technologies, they can delay the entry of affordable generics and biosimilars. Voluntary licensing, patent pools, and flexibilities in international trade agreements can be used to expand access while still providing incentives for research. Some advocates call for new models altogether, such as prize funds, public–private partnerships, or open science frameworks that decouple profits from high per-patient prices. Whatever the mechanism, the underlying ethical question remains: how do we fairly reward creativity and investment without allowing the ability to pay to determine who lives and who dies.

Community engagement and co-design are essential if biotech is to serve diverse populations equitably. Too often, technologies are developed with minimal input from those who will use them, leading to tools that are ill-suited to local needs, beliefs, or constraints. For example, a genetic screening program that does not consider cultural views on disability or kinship may provoke resistance or harm. A diagnostic test that requires refrigeration or complex sample handling may be unusable in many clinics.

Involving local health workers, patient groups, and community leaders from the earliest stages of design can surface these issues before they become barriers. It also helps ensure that benefits are defined not only in terms of abstract clinical outcomes, but in terms of what actually matters to people's lives.

Global health emergencies expose the biotech divide with brutal clarity. During outbreaks and pandemics, vaccines, diagnostics, and treatments are often developed at unprecedented speed—but their distribution follows familiar patterns. Wealthy countries may secure supplies far beyond their immediate needs, while others wait months or years. Manufacturing capacity clustered in a few regions becomes a bottleneck, and export controls can hinder global solidarity. These dynamics reveal that access is not just about scientific capability; it is about political will, international cooperation, and the structures of global trade. After each crisis, calls for fairer systems grow louder, but reforms are often partial and short-lived. Building truly equitable biotech access requires learning from these moments and locking in changes before attention wanes.

Measurement matters in efforts to close the divide. Without data on who is receiving advanced therapies and who is not, inequities can remain invisible or be dismissed as anecdotal. Collecting and analyzing access metrics—broken down by region, income, race, gender, and other relevant factors—allows policymakers and advocates to track progress and hold systems accountable. Transparency about pricing, trial locations, and licensing agreements can also shine light on structural barriers. Of course, data alone do not guarantee change; they must be paired with advocacy, policy interventions, and community organizing. Still, without clear evidence, it is easy for the benefits of biotech to be overestimated and their uneven distribution underestimated.

Education and health literacy are quiet but powerful tools for narrowing the biotech gap. People who understand basic concepts about genetics, risk, and clinical trials are better equipped to make informed decisions, ask questions, and advocate for themselves. At the same time, professionals trained in culturally responsive care and aware of global disparities are more likely to notice when patterns of exclusion arise. Education must be adapted to local languages, metaphors, and concerns, rather than imported wholesale. It should also be reciprocal: experts have much to learn from community knowledge about health practices, priorities, and barriers. When dialogue flows both ways, biotech can be integrated into care in ways that respect local wisdom rather than displacing it.

There is a temptation, especially in high-tech fields, to assume that innovation itself will eventually trickle down and benefit everyone. History suggests otherwise. Without policies aimed explicitly at equity, new technologies often increase inequality, at least in the short and medium term. Those with resources, connections, and political influence adopt them first, gaining additional advantages. In health, this can mean that the healthiest and wealthiest live even longer and better, while preventable illness continues elsewhere. Confronting this requires moving equity from the margins to the center of biotech planning. Questions like "Who will have access," "What will this cost," and "How will this affect existing disparities" need to be asked at the beginning of research programs, not as an afterthought once products are ready to launch.

At the same time, it is important to recognize and celebrate successes where the divide has narrowed. Global efforts to expand access to antiretroviral therapy for HIV, to distribute vaccines for childhood diseases, and to combat neglected tropical diseases have saved millions of lives across income levels. These achievements were not inevitable; they required activism, international funding mechanisms, generics production, and sustained political pressure. They provide models for how biotech benefits can be shared more widely, even when initial conditions are unequal. Learning from these experiences means examining not only the scientific advances, but also the coalitions and policies that made them accessible.

Ultimately, access and equity in biotechnology are not technical problems with purely technical solutions. They are questions about what kind of world we want to build with the tools we have. We can choose to treat advanced therapies as luxury goods, available to a few, or as public goods that societies strive to share as broadly as possible. We can organize research agendas around the diseases of those who can pay the most, or around the burdens that cause the most suffering, regardless of market size. We can design systems that assume scarcity and competition, or we can experiment with models rooted in solidarity and shared benefit. None of these choices are simple, and all involve trade-offs. But they are choices, not fate.

In the context of this book, the global biotech divide is the ground on which all other chapters stand. Gene editing, regenerative medicine, immunotherapies, synthetic biology, AI diagnostics—each holds immense promise, yet each can deepen or diminish inequality depending on how it is governed and distributed. As we move next into questions of regulation, risk, and responsibility, the themes of access and equity should remain in view. Laws, policies, and safety frameworks do more than keep people safe from immediate harms; they also shape who is included in the benefits of innovation and who is left waiting outside the door.

Chapter .18

Regulators, Risk, and Responsibility

Laws, policies, and safety frameworks guide, enable, and constrain biotech innovation.

Every powerful technology forces society to answer a quiet but urgent question: who is responsible for making sure this does more good than harm. In biotechnology, that question shows up in consent forms, drug approval processes, lab rules, and international agreements that most people never see. It shows up in checklists before a clinical trial, in audits of manufacturing plants, and in the debates of regulatory agencies deciding whether a therapy is ready for wider use. Regulation is sometimes portrayed as a brake on progress, but it is just as much a steering wheel and a guardrail. Without it, innovation can veer into exploitation or catastrophe; with it, innovation may move more slowly but on a course that earns public trust. Risk is not something we can eliminate from biotech, but it is something we can share, shape, and plan for.

At its core, regulation tries to answer three questions: is this safe enough, does it work well enough, and is it being used fairly enough. The answers are never simple yes or no; they are judgment calls based on incomplete evidence, evolving science, and diverse values. Drug agencies weigh data from preclinical studies, animal models, and human trials, looking for patterns of benefit and harm. Ethics committees assess whether people enrolling in studies understand what they are agreeing to, and whether the trial design respects their rights. Environmental and agricultural authorities consider how engineered organisms might spread or affect ecosystems. None of these decisions happen in a vacuum; they are influenced by public pressure, political priorities, and economic interests. Responsibility, in this context, is distributed across many actors, which makes coordination both essential and difficult.

Biotech's risk landscape is unusual because it spans multiple timescales and levels of impact. Some risks are immediate and personal: an unexpected immune reaction to a gene therapy, a rare but serious side effect of a biologic drug, a lab worker exposed to a pathogen. Others are slower and more diffuse: gradual erosion of antibiotic effectiveness, accumulation of off-target genetic changes that only manifest years later, or subtle ecological disruptions from releasing engineered organisms. Still others are societal and ethical: shifts in norms about disability, privacy invasions through genomic databases, and widening inequality as advanced therapies reach only a few. When regulators and policymakers talk about "risk," they are trying to hold all these dimensions in mind at once. The challenge is that different stakeholders experience and prioritize these risks differently, depending on where they sit.

Historically, many of the frameworks that govern biotech grew out of earlier crises. Public outrage over unethical experiments and abuses in research led to principles emphasizing respect for persons, beneficence, and justice in human studies. High-profile tragedies in gene therapy, blood products, and drug safety prompted stricter oversight of clinical trials, manufacturing, and post-market surveillance. Each painful episode left behind a layer of rules designed to prevent repetition. This history can make regulation feel reactive and patchwork, but it also means that many safety standards are written in the language of lessons learned. The responsibility of current practitioners is to honor those lessons without treating them as static, recognizing that new technologies may require updated guardrails rather than simply wedging them into old molds.

Preclinical and clinical testing are among the most visible expressions of biotech regulation. Before a therapy reaches human volunteers, it must be evaluated in cell systems and animal models for toxicity, dosing, and mechanism of action. These studies are imperfect predictors of human outcomes, but they are designed to catch glaring problems early. Once a therapy enters human trials, the process unfolds in stages, from small safety-focused studies to larger trials assessing efficacy and comparative benefit. Regulators review plans, monitor emerging data, and sometimes halt studies when concerns arise. Researchers have their own responsibilities: to report results honestly, including negative and ambiguous findings; to stop or adjust trials when risks outweigh benefits; and to ensure that participants are not misled by hype. Science, ethics, and law intersect in these decisions, and none of them can be safely ignored.

Manufacturing and quality control are quieter but no less crucial arenas of responsibility. A therapy that works beautifully in a small trial can become dangerous if production is inconsistent, contaminated, or poorly documented. Biologics and cell therapies, in particular, are sensitive to variations in process; slight shifts in temperature, equipment, or raw materials can alter their behavior. Regulatory agencies require detailed manufacturing plans, batch testing, and traceability systems that track ingredients from source to patient. This can seem bureaucratic, but it is central to ensuring that what leaves a factory or cell-processing lab is what the label claims. When errors happen—a contaminated line, a mislabeled dose—the results can be severe for patients and for trust in the entire field. Responsibility here is as much about routine vigilance as it is about dramatic decision points.

Gene editing and gene drive technologies have prompted regulators to rethink traditional boundaries between medical and environmental oversight. Editing cells inside a single patient's body is one kind of risk; releasing an engineered mosquito that can spread a genetic trait through a wild population is another entirely. The former is largely governed by clinical and drug regulations, focusing on individual consent and safety. The latter requires ecological modeling, community consultation, and regional or global agreements, because the effects could cross borders and generations. Risk in such cases includes not only what we can quantify in models, but also what we cannot yet foresee. Responsibility means acknowledging uncertainty explicitly, designing reversibility where possible, and setting criteria for when to pause or stop interventions that behave unexpectedly.

Data governance sits at the crossroads of biotech and digital regulation. Genomic databases, electronic health records, and sensor streams power AI models, stratified medicine, and public health surveillance. But they also create vulnerabilities: the possibility that sensitive information could be hacked, re-identified, or used for purposes never consented to. Regulators and lawmakers must decide who owns these data, who can access them, under what conditions, and with what oversight. Companies and researchers have corresponding responsibilities to implement strong security, minimize data collection to what is truly needed, and be transparent about how data contribute to profits or products. Individuals, too, face decisions about what to share and with whom, often without full visibility into the consequences. A responsible data framework tries to avoid placing all the burden on users while leaving systems opaque and asymmetric.

International coordination is both necessary and fragile in biotech regulation. Viruses, data, and know-how cross borders much more easily than laws do. A therapy banned in one country may be developed in another with looser rules. A data center in one jurisdiction may store information collected from people worldwide. Germline editing, synthetic pathogens, and cross-species chimeras are examples of technologies that many argue require global norms, not just national ones. International organizations, scientific academies, and cross-border working groups can articulate shared principles and voluntary standards, but enforcement is often weak. Responsibility in this arena involves peer pressure, transparency, and the professional culture of science as much as formal law. Researchers and companies can choose to abide by higher standards than the minimum required, signaling that ethical commitments are not optional extras.

Regulation must also contend with speed: the urgency of unmet medical needs, the rapid pace of discovery, and the commercial incentives to be first. Patients with life-threatening conditions may be willing to accept higher levels of risk and uncertainty for a chance at benefit, pressing regulators to accelerate approval pathways. Programs that allow early access to promising therapies, conditional approvals based on surrogate endpoints, and rolling review of data are all attempts to balance speed with caution. Yet there is a danger that, under pressure, standards erode slowly, making it harder to distinguish genuine breakthroughs from marginal or unproven interventions. Responsibility here involves honesty about what is known and unknown, clear commitments to follow-up studies, and mechanisms to withdraw or modify approvals when real-world data contradict early optimism.

Companies play a central role in biotech risk and responsibility, because they often control development pipelines, marketing strategies, and pricing. Their decisions influence not only who has access, as discussed in the previous chapter, but also how aggressively products are promoted and how negative results are handled. Regulatory frameworks attempt to align company incentives with public health through requirements for post-market surveillance, penalties for misleading advertising, and obligations to report adverse events. Shareholders and boards also hold power, as they set expectations for returns that can either support long-term, careful development or push toward shortcuts and risky bets. Corporate responsibility in biotech includes not only compliance with laws, but also internal cultures that value integrity, transparency, and patient welfare.

Public engagement is increasingly recognized as part of responsible governance, not a public relations afterthought. Communities affected by new technologies—whether through clinical use, environmental release, or data collection—have perspectives that technical experts alone cannot provide. Their concerns may range from safety and access to cultural meaning and historical context. When regulators and developers involve the public early and genuinely, through consultations, citizen panels, or partnerships, they often discover issues that scientific risk assessments did not capture. They also build legitimacy for decisions, even controversial ones, because people feel heard rather than managed. Responsibility here is two-sided: institutions must create real opportunities for input, and participants must be willing to engage with complex trade-offs rather than demand impossible perfection.

Communication about risk may be the most delicate responsibility of all. When something goes wrong—a trial halted for safety, an adverse reaction in a patient, a data breach—it can be tempting to minimize or spin the story to protect reputations. Yet trust is more often damaged by secrecy than by frank admission of problems. Clear, timely, and compassionate communication that explains what happened, what is being done, and what is still uncertain can maintain or even strengthen public confidence. The same holds for communicating risk before decisions are made. People need to understand that no therapy is without downsides, that side effects can exist alongside benefits, and that "zero risk" is not a realistic goal. Mature regulation treats the public as capable of understanding nuance, not as an audience to be shielded from complexity.

There is an important distinction between individual risk and systemic risk in biotechnology. An individual may accept a high chance of side effects for a personally meaningful chance at benefit; that is their choice in consultation with clinicians. Systemic risk, however, involves consequences that fall on others who did not choose them: antibiotic resistance driven by overuse, erosion of privacy norms through unregulated data sharing, ecological shifts after release of engineered organisms. Regulators and policymakers have a duty to protect against these broader harms, even when individuals or companies are willing to take the gamble. This can mean saying no to certain applications altogether, or setting conditions that feel frustratingly conservative to innovators. The tension between personal autonomy and collective protection is not new, but biotech gives it sharper edges.

Unregulated or loosely regulated spaces in biotech raise special concerns. These include offshore clinics offering unproven stem cell or gene therapies, "wellness" products that blur the line with medical claims, and gray-market genetic modification kits. People drawn to such offerings are often those who feel failed or ignored by mainstream systems, making them vulnerable to exploitation. Regulatory agencies can issue warnings, pursue enforcement actions, and collaborate across borders to shut down the most egregious operations. But they also need to ask why demand for these services exists and how to better integrate evidence-based innovation into accessible, humane care. Simply cracking down without addressing underlying desperation risks driving risky practices further underground. Responsibility extends beyond policing; it includes building systems that reduce the appeal of dangerous shortcuts.

Within research and clinical practice, professional norms act as an invisible layer of regulation. Codes of conduct, peer review, and community expectations can discourage reckless experiments even when laws are silent. Whistleblower protections and avenues for raising concerns internally are part of this ecosystem, allowing people to speak up when they see corners being cut or data being distorted. Mentorship and training that emphasize ethical reflection alongside technical skill help build a culture where responsibility is shared, not outsourced. When scandals do arise, how institutions respond—by silencing critics or by investigating and correcting problems—sends a message about what really matters. In this sense, regulation is as much about character and culture as it is about statutes and guidelines.

Looking ahead, the regulatory landscape will need to adapt continuously as biotechnologies converge and hybridize. A single intervention might combine gene editing, engineered cells, AI-driven dosing algorithms, and remote monitoring devices. Traditional regulatory silos—drugs here, devices there, software in another corner—may not map cleanly onto such integrated products. New frameworks will need to consider systems as wholes, evaluating how their parts interact in real-world use. They will also need to be flexible enough to accommodate iterative updates, especially in digital components, without compromising safety. The temptation will be to either overcomplicate the rules or to declare existing categories "good enough"; responsibility lies in doing the harder work of thoughtful redesign.

In the larger story of this book, regulators, risk, and responsibility form the connective tissue that holds biotech's ambitions in relationship with society's values. Without them, chapters about gene therapy, synthetic biology, AI, and at-home diagnostics would describe technologies floating free of accountability. With them, those chapters become parts of a negotiated social project: an ongoing attempt to harness biological power for healing while respecting autonomy, equity, and the environment. As we move next to biotech in everyday life, beyond clinics and labs, the questions of who bears risk and who takes responsibility will follow us into supermarkets, farms, workplaces, and homes. The frameworks we build now will shape not only what is allowed, but what feels acceptable as biology and technology intertwine more deeply with daily experience.

Chapter .19

Biotech in Everyday Life

Biotechnology is increasingly shaping our food, environment, and daily experiences beyond traditional medicine.

Biotechnology often seems most visible in hospitals and research labs, but its fingerprints are all over everyday life. It is present in the bread that rises on a kitchen counter, the detergent that lifts stains in cold water, and the cheese on a pizza. Yeasts, bacteria, and engineered enzymes quietly work behind the scenes to make products more efficient, longer lasting, or easier to manufacture. Many of these uses build on age-old practices like fermentation, now tuned with modern genetics and precision control. Others are entirely new, born from synthetic biology and industrial bioengineering. When we look closely, it becomes clear that biotech is not a distant field; it is part of the ordinary routines that fill our days.

Food and agriculture are perhaps the most obvious places where biotech intersects with everyday experience. Crops have long been selectively bred for yield, flavor, and resilience, but newer tools allow targeted changes to specific genes. Plants can be engineered to resist pests, tolerate drought, or use nutrients more efficiently, potentially reducing reliance on chemical pesticides and fertilizers. These traits can help stabilize harvests in the face of climate uncertainty and population growth. At the same time, concerns about ecological impact, corporate control, and labeling have made genetically modified foods a recurring public debate. Walking through a supermarket, we are often encountering these technologies whether or not they are explicitly marked.

Biotech also shapes what happens after food leaves the field. Enzymes derived from microbes are used in baking to improve texture, extend shelf life, and keep bread soft for longer. In brewing and winemaking, carefully selected yeast strains influence not only fermentation speed but also flavor profiles and aroma. Dairy products rely on cultures that have been refined over generations, with some now produced using engineered microbes that create specific proteins or flavors. Meat alternatives increasingly use plant proteins or fermentation-derived ingredients that mimic the taste and mouthfeel of animal products. For many consumers, the sensory experience is familiar, even if the production methods have grown more sophisticated and less visible.

Genetically modified crops and ingredients have sparked intense discussions about safety and ethics. Large scientific reviews have generally found that approved genetically modified foods are as safe to eat as their conventional counterparts, yet public suspicion persists in many places. Part of this tension arises from issues of trust: trust in regulatory agencies, in corporations that develop seeds, and in the transparency of labeling. People may accept biotech in medicine while feeling uneasy about it in food, where cultural meaning and identity are deeply involved. The conversation is often less about the specific genes involved and more about who controls the food system and whose values shape it. Everyday choices at the grocery store thus carry echoes of broader questions about power and participation in technology.

Biotechnology extends beyond crops to the animals that share our lives and diets. Selective breeding has long shaped livestock, but genetic tools now allow more direct alterations. Animals may be engineered to be more resistant to disease, to grow more efficiently, or to produce milk or eggs with altered nutritional profiles. Some projects aim to reduce environmental impact by creating animals that emit less methane or require less feed. Others focus on welfare, such as pigs bred without certain traits that cause distress. These efforts sit at the intersection of compassion, productivity, and unease about designing living beings for human purposes.

The rise of cultivated meat introduces another layer to everyday biotech. In this approach, animal cells are grown in bioreactors instead of animals being raised and slaughtered. Muscle and fat cells are nourished with carefully formulated media, encouraged to form tissues that resemble traditional meat in taste and texture. For consumers, the idea of eating meat without killing animals can be appealing, but the methods can also feel unfamiliar or unsettling. Questions arise about energy use, cost, and whether such products will genuinely reduce environmental and ethical burdens. When cultivated meat appears on menus or in stores, it will bring these abstract debates into literal bite-sized form.

Industrial biotechnology plays a large, mostly invisible role in household products. Enzymes used in laundry detergents help break down stains at lower temperatures, saving energy and protecting fabrics. In dishwashing liquids and cleaners, bio-based surfactants and catalysts can reduce the need for harsh chemicals or high heat. Many of these ingredients are produced by engineered microbes that ferment sugar or other feedstocks into useful compounds. This is sometimes described as a shift from petrochemical factories to biorefineries. People rarely think about these details while loading a washing machine, yet they are interacting with biotech every time the cycle starts.

Bioplastics and bio-based materials represent another everyday touchpoint. Some packaging, utensils, and textiles now incorporate polymers derived from plant sugars or other biological sources rather than fossil fuels. These materials can, in some cases, be compostable or more easily recyclable, though real-world performance varies. Synthetic biology allows designers to tweak the properties of these materials, adjusting flexibility, durability, or transparency. The hope is to reduce reliance on non-renewable resources and lower the environmental footprint of disposable goods. However, the success of such efforts depends on infrastructure, consumer behavior, and honest communication about what "bio-based" actually means in practice.

Environmental biotechnology reaches beyond products into the spaces where we live and work. Microbes are used in wastewater treatment plants to break down organic matter and contaminants, quietly protecting rivers and oceans. Some industrial facilities use biofilters, packed with specialized bacteria, to remove odors and pollutants from air emissions. There are projects where engineered organisms capture heavy metals from contaminated soils or break down toxic chemicals into less harmful forms. These applications seldom appear on product labels, yet they help determine whether the air is breathable and the water is safe. Everyday environmental quality is, in part, a result of these unseen bio-based processes.

Biotech also shapes the energy that powers daily life. Fermentation-based production of biofuels, such as ethanol and biodiesel, has been part of energy systems for years. Newer approaches engineer microbes to convert waste gases, agricultural residues, or even carbon dioxide into fuels or chemical feedstocks. While biofuels alone cannot solve the energy transition, they can complement other renewable sources, especially in sectors that are hard to electrify. The impact shows up in transportation, where blends of biofuel and conventional fuel run cars, buses, and planes. Filling a tank or boarding a flight may involve biotech-derived energy, even if it is not prominently advertised.

Personal care products also enlist biotech in subtle ways. Shampoos, soaps, and cosmetics sometimes contain ingredients produced via fermentation rather than animal extraction or synthetic chemistry. Hyaluronic acid for skin care, for example, can be made by engineered microbes instead of being harvested from animal tissue. Fragrance components may be brewed in vats rather than distilled from large quantities of plants, reducing land and resource use. Some brands promote these methods as more sustainable or ethical, while others simply incorporate them quietly. Consumers may notice softer textures or different scents without realizing that microbes played a role in the formulation.

Biotech is present in pets' lives as well. Vaccines, parasite treatments, and improved diagnostics are direct extensions of medical biotechnology into veterinary care. Pet foods increasingly use insights from microbiome research and nutrition science to adjust formulations for gut health or specific conditions. There are even experimental projects exploring cultivated meat or insect-based proteins for pet diets, aiming to reduce the environmental impact of traditional animal feed. For many people, the health and comfort of companion animals are emotionally important, so the adoption of biotech in this realm can feel deeply personal. It is another way that advanced biology shows up not just in abstract policy, but in relationships with living beings we love.

Biotechnology influences the built environment in more experimental but growing ways. Designers and architects explore bio-based materials such as mycelium composites, where fungal networks grow into shapes that can serve as insulation, packaging, or even structural elements. Algae bioreactors have been integrated into building facades to capture carbon and generate biomass. Living walls and green roofs, while not always high tech, embody a similar principle of integrating life into structures for temperature regulation and air quality. As these ideas mature, homes and workplaces may become sites where engineered life forms are intentionally embedded as functional components, not just decorations.

Education and entertainment are beginning to incorporate biotech themes more directly. Science museums host interactive exhibits about genomics, synthetic biology, and microbiomes, often allowing visitors to visualize their own cells or DNA. Comics, films, and novels regularly feature gene editing, biohacking, and engineered organisms as plot elements, shaping public imagination. Some citizen science projects invite people to swab their environments, grow microbes on plates, and observe the diversity of life around them. These experiences make biotechnology feel less like an abstract discipline and more like a set of tangible processes that anyone can observe and question.

They also subtly influence how people respond to real-world biotech debates.

Do-it-yourself biology spaces, mentioned earlier, are another everyday manifestation of biotech's spread. Community labs offer workshops where people learn to pipette, culture bacteria, and run simple genetic experiments using safe strains. Participants may be students, artists, hobbyists, or professionals from other fields. These spaces can demystify laboratory practices and give people a sense of agency, showing that biology is not only the domain of large institutions. At the same time, they raise questions about safety, oversight, and equity in access to scientific tools. A world where some neighborhoods have vibrant community labs while others lack basic science education could reinforce existing divides.

Marketing often uses biotech language to influence everyday choices. Phrases like "bio-based," "natural," "GMO-free," and "probiotic" appear on labels, sometimes with clear meaning and sometimes as vague appeals. Products may be advertised as harnessing the power of microbes or plant-derived technology, even when the underlying science is modest. Conversely, items may proudly proclaim the absence of certain biotechnologies, responding to consumer concerns or trends. This environment can be confusing, because scientific nuance is condensed into slogans and symbols. Learning to read these claims critically becomes part of everyday media literacy in a biotech-shaped world.

Biotech's role in environmental monitoring affects daily life indirectly but significantly. Sensors and assays based on molecular techniques detect contaminants in water supplies, track harmful algal blooms, and monitor pathogens in sewage. These tools help authorities issue boil-water advisories, close beaches when necessary, and respond to outbreaks more quickly. During disease surges, wastewater analysis can provide early warnings about rising infection levels in communities. Residents may never know that such testing guided public health decisions, but they experience the outcomes in advisories, school notices, and policy changes. The safety of everyday activities like drinking tap water or swimming in lakes is entwined with these biological surveillance systems.

Biotech is also shaping how we think about waste and circular economies. Microbes are used to break down organic waste into biogas or fertilizers, turning food scraps and agricultural residues into energy and soil amendments. Some research focuses on organisms that can degrade plastics or convert waste streams into valuable chemicals. Community composting programs, even when low tech, rely on microbial activity to transform leftovers into rich soil. When people sort their trash, separate organics, or use compostable packaging, they are participating in processes that depend on biological transformation. Everyday waste routines become part of larger biotechnological cycles.

In workplaces, biotech appears in safety protocols, materials, and health programs. Offices and factories may use air purifiers that incorporate bio-based filters or coatings, though these are often marketed simply as advanced filtration. Corporate wellness programs might include microbiome-informed nutrition advice or genetic risk assessments offered as benefits. Some workplaces handle biological materials directly, from food production to pharmaceutical manufacturing, turning biotech into an ordinary part of daily tasks for many employees. Even in jobs far from the lab, interactions with bio-derived materials and health technologies are increasingly common.

Biotech's presence in everyday life can create a sense of both comfort and vulnerability. On one hand, it is reassuring to know that food safety testing, water quality monitoring, and disease surveillance are bolstered by advanced tools. On the other hand, dependence on complex systems can feel unsettling, especially when they are not transparent. People may worry about hidden risks, data misuse, or unintended ecological consequences. The challenge is to build systems that are not only effective but also accountable and understandable, so that everyday reliance on biotech does not feel like blind trust in invisible processes.

Cultural responses to biotech in daily life are diverse. Some communities embrace fermented foods, herbal remedies, and traditional practices as forms of low-tech biotechnology rooted in heritage. Others are drawn to cutting-edge products that promise efficiency, sustainability, or novelty. The boundaries between "traditional" and "modern" biology are often fuzzier than they appear; many age-old practices can now be explained in molecular terms. Recognizing this continuity can soften the sense that biotech is an alien force invading daily life. It can also highlight the importance of respecting and learning from longstanding ecological knowledge as new tools are developed.

Ethical questions accompany biotech in everyday contexts just as they do in medicine. Who benefits from increased yields in agriculture, and who bears the risks of environmental change. How are communities consulted when engineered organisms are deployed in their surroundings. Which workers are exposed to new materials and processes, and are they protected and fairly compensated. These questions are not limited to large policy arenas; they show up in local zoning meetings, school board discussions, and neighborhood organizing. The ethical shape of everyday biotech emerges from countless small decisions as much as from grand public debates.

Education and public dialogue are essential for navigating biotech's everyday presence. People do not need to master every technical detail, but they benefit from understanding basic concepts like genes, microbes, and risk. Schools, media, and community organizations can help build this literacy through engaging, context-rich learning rather than abstract lectures. When people can connect scientific ideas to their own experience—why bread rises, how vaccines work, what compost does—they are better prepared to interpret biotech claims and participate in decisions. Everyday understanding becomes a form of shared power in a technologically saturated world.

Ultimately, biotech in everyday life invites a reframing of how we see our relationship with the living world. Instead of viewing biology as something that happens only in bodies or distant ecosystems, we can recognize it in kitchens, gardens, factories, and city streets. Our choices about what to eat, what to wear, how to clean, and how to travel are entangled with biological processes that extend far beyond our immediate view. Recognizing this entanglement does not mean living in constant scrutiny or fear. It means acknowledging that we are participants in a web of designed and natural life, and that our daily habits help steer how that web evolves.

In the context of this book, biotech in everyday life serves as a reminder that the most transformative technologies are not always the ones that make headlines. They are often the ones that quietly become normal, folded into routines until they feel unremarkable. The enzymes in laundry detergent, the microbes in waste treatment, and the sensors in air and water systems are as much a part of the biotech revolution as headline-grabbing gene edits. As we turn to the final chapter on the next decades of medicine, it is worth carrying this insight forward: the future will not arrive only in dramatic interventions in hospitals, but also in the subtle shifts that change how we live, eat, move, and care for the world around us.

Chapter .20

The Next 50 Years of Medicine

Biology is becoming programmable, opening futures in which medicine is transformed yet again.

Looking ahead half a century can feel like staring into a fog, but some shapes are already visible. The core shift driving future medicine is the idea that biology is becoming programmable, much like early computers once did. Instead of treating the body as a black box that occasionally breaks, we are beginning to understand it as a dynamic, information-rich system that can be measured, modeled, and adjusted. Genes, cells, and microbiomes are no longer just observed; they are edited, engineered, and guided. The coming decades will not be about a single "miracle cure," but about layering many of these technologies into a more responsive, personalized, and preventive kind of care. The question is not only what we will be able to do, but how we will choose to use that power.

One of the most profound changes will likely be the shift from treatment to prediction and prevention. Instead of waiting for a heart attack or stroke, medicine will increasingly estimate your risks based on genetics, biomarkers, behavior, environment, and patterns in continuous data. Smart diagnostics, wearables, and home tests will feed streams of information into models that recognize early warning signs long before symptoms appear. Clinics may feel less like places to "fix what broke" and more like hubs that help people adjust course in time. This does not mean that disease disappears, but that many crises could be replaced by earlier, quieter interventions. The art of medicine will be as much about coaching and fine-tuning as about rescue.

Genomic information will likely be woven into routine care from birth onward. Newborn screening may expand from a handful of biochemical tests to comprehensive genomic panels that identify serious, actionable risks early. As people age, periodic updates to their risk profiles—based on both inherited variants and acquired changes—could guide screening, lifestyle advice, and preventive therapies. For some conditions, gene editing or gene silencing might be offered before disease fully develops, nudging biology away from harmful trajectories. The challenge will be to handle this information without turning life into a constant risk report, or making people feel defined by probabilities rather than possibilities. Medicine will need to develop not just better tests, but better ways to talk about what they mean.

Cell and gene therapies are likely to become more refined, more targeted, and more common. Techniques that are now reserved for rare diseases and aggressive cancers may broaden to address more prevalent conditions, such as heart failure, arthritis, or neurodegeneration. Delivery systems will improve, making it easier to send genetic payloads to specific tissues without triggering dangerous immune responses. Ex vivo approaches—editing cells outside the body and reinfusing them—may be complemented by in vivo editing that can be done with an infusion or injection. As safety profiles become clearer and manufacturing becomes more scalable, the question will shift from "Can we do this at all" to "Whom should we treat, when, and with what goals."

Regenerative medicine will likely move from small, tightly controlled trials to more routine procedures in certain fields. Bioengineered tissues for skin, cartilage, and perhaps segments of blood vessels or airways may become standard options in surgery. Stem-cell–derived cells could be used to repair damaged heart muscle after a heart attack or to replace specific neuron populations in selected neurological diseases. Organoids grown from a person's own cells may help test which drugs or combinations work best before clinicians commit to a course of therapy. Not every organ will be replaceable, and not every damage will be reversible, but the vocabulary of "irreversible" may shrink. Rehabilitation might be paired more often with regeneration, turning recovery into a collaboration between biology and engineering.

Immunotherapies will continue to spread beyond oncology into autoimmune diseases, allergies, chronic infections, and even some forms of organ rejection. We may see more therapies that retrain the immune system toward tolerance where it is overactive and vigilance where it is exhausted. Personalized cancer vaccines, designed from the specific mutations in a patient's tumor, could become part of standard care in many malignancies. At the same time, off-the-shelf engineered cell therapies might be readily available in pharmacies or hospitals, reducing waiting times and costs. The immune system will be seen less as something to suppress or boost in rough ways and more as a programmable network to be tuned. Managing that tuning wisely will be an ongoing responsibility.

The microbiome will probably be treated less like a mysterious black box and more like a cultivable garden. Future therapies may include precise microbial consortia tailored to individual needs, replacing broad probiotics with targeted "microbial prescriptions." Engineered microbes could sense inflammation, metabolic disturbances, or toxins and respond by producing beneficial molecules exactly where they are needed. Diet, environment, and microbiome-directed drugs will form a triangle of influence, with clinicians helping people adjust each corner. We will likely come to see some chronic diseases as disturbances of ecosystems within us rather than just failures of human cells. Caring for those ecosystems will be part of everyday health practice.

Artificial intelligence will be deeply embedded in nearly every stage of medicine, often in ways that are no longer separately noticed. In research, AI-driven models will help design molecules, simulate clinical trials, and integrate insights across millions of papers and datasets. In clinics, decision-support systems will summarize histories, suggest diagnoses, and propose treatment options, presenting clinicians with reasoned, explainable recommendations rather than opaque verdicts. In homes, AI companions may help people interpret their health data, remind them about medications, and flag when something needs professional attention. The central issue will not be whether AI is used, but whether it is used fairly, transparently, and under human guidance that keeps responsibility clear.

Smart diagnostics and wearables will likely become less obtrusive and more integrated into the fabric of life. Clothing may include sensors that track posture, movement, and physiology without requiring separate devices. Home environments could monitor air quality, noise, and sleep patterns, suggesting adjustments for comfort and health. For some conditions, digital biomarkers—patterns in speech, typing, walking, or social activity—might help detect early cognitive decline, mood shifts, or relapse risk. People will have opportunities to know much more about their bodies than previous generations ever could. The key question will be how to prevent this from turning into a relentless self-surveillance that erodes peace of mind.

Mental health care will probably be transformed by a combination of biological insights and digital tools. Advances in neurobiology, genetics, and immunology may reveal distinct subtypes of conditions now lumped under broad labels like "depression" or "schizophrenia." Biomarkers and imaging may help guide more precise medication choices and non-pharmacologic interventions. Digital therapeutics, virtual reality exposures, and AI-guided coaching may augment traditional therapy, expanding access to support in places where clinicians are scarce. At the same time, societies will need to confront the mental health impacts of living in constantly connected, data-rich environments. Technology will be both part of the solution and part of the problem, demanding careful attention to how it shapes attention, relationships, and rest.

Global health will be influenced by biotechnology in ways that could either narrow or widen inequities. In optimistic scenarios, affordable diagnostics, vaccines, and therapies produced through scalable bioengineering will reach more people through strengthened health systems and regional manufacturing. Data-sharing networks may help identify outbreaks early and coordinate responses, using genomic surveillance and wastewater monitoring as routine tools. However, without strong commitments to equity, advanced therapies may cluster in wealthy regions while others see little benefit. The next fifty years of medicine will be judged not only by what is technically possible, but by how evenly its fruits are shared. The global biotech divide is not a peripheral issue; it is a central test of our collective priorities.

Regulation and ethics will have to evolve in step with biotechnology's growing capabilities. Static rulebooks cannot keep pace with living, learning systems that update themselves or treatments that permanently alter biology. Regulatory frameworks will likely become more adaptive, using real-world evidence, continuous monitoring, and tiered risk models to guide decisions. Citizens may play a more direct role in shaping policies through assemblies and participatory processes, especially around germline editing, environmental releases, and data governance. The next half-century will require not only clever scientists, but also thoughtful ethicists, policymakers, and engaged publics who can navigate trade-offs with nuance. The legitimacy of future medicine will rest on this shared governance as much as on technical performance.

Longevity science and aging interventions will almost certainly be a major frontier. Therapies that modestly slow aging processes, clear senescent cells, or support tissue repair could add healthy years for many people. If used wisely and fairly, these tools might compress morbidity, allowing more people to remain active and independent later into life. If used narrowly and expensively, they could become status markers that widen gaps in health and wealth. Societies will need to rethink work, retirement, education, and intergenerational solidarity if significant extensions of healthspan become common. Medicine will not only be about saving lives, but about shaping the texture and timing of whole lifetimes.

The boundary between medical and everyday biotechnology will continue to blur. Personalized nutrition, sleep optimization, cognitive enhancement, and mood modulation will be sold through a mixture of regulated therapies and wellness products. Some people will embrace a highly quantified approach to life, tracking metrics for performance and longevity; others will seek simpler, less monitored paths. The cultural conversation about what is "normal," what is "good enough," and what is worth changing will grow more complex. Medicine will need to honor a range of choices, including the choice to decline certain interventions, without pathologizing people who do not chase every optimization.

Education will be a crucial foundation for navigating the next fifty years of medicine. Basic literacy in genetics, risk, data, and ethics will help people understand options and ask informed questions. Health professionals will need fluency in technology and humility about uncertainty. Scientific training will need to emphasize collaboration across disciplines and engagement with communities, not just technical prowess. In many places, this will mean expanding access to quality education long before any biotech therapy is administered. The future of medicine will depend as much on schools and public discourse as on labs and clinics.

Amid all these changes, some constants will remain. People will still fear, hope, grieve, and love. They will still sit in exam rooms with worries that have no simple answers, and they will still weigh trade-offs between side effects and benefits. No matter how sophisticated tools become, someone will need to listen carefully, explain kindly, and stand alongside patients in uncertainty. The human relationship at the heart of medicine will not disappear; if anything, it may become more important as technologies grow more complex and abstract. Compassion, trust, and presence are not made obsolete by progress; they are what make progress bearable and meaningful.

The next fifty years of medicine will likely not feel like a single revolution, but like a series of overlapping shifts that gradually become part of normal life. A child born into a world of genomic screening, smart diagnostics, and regenerative options will not experience them as miracles, but as the background of what care looks like. Our task, in the present, is to shape that background with foresight and care. We cannot predict every discovery or crisis, but we can set trajectories: toward equity rather than exclusion, toward transparency rather than secrecy, toward support rather than surveillance. In that sense, the future of medicine is less something that happens to us and more something we collectively write.

In the story this book has told, biotechnology has moved from decoding the human blueprint to rewriting it, from patching bodies to regenerating tissues, from generic drugs to personalized interventions, from hospitals to homes and everyday life. The next fifty years will continue that trajectory, deepening the programmability of biology while testing our ability to govern it wisely. The question that echoes through each chapter is simple and demanding: with all this new power, who will we choose to be.

Author Reflection – The Next 50 Years of Medicine

Writing this final chapter, I felt a tug-of-war between excitement and humility. On one side is the genuine wonder at what might be possible: diseases tamed before they take hold, tissues repaired that once stayed broken, lives extended with more years of clarity and connection. On the other side is the awareness that technology alone has never guaranteed justice, kindness, or wisdom. We have had powerful tools before and used them in ways that both healed and harmed. What stays with me most is the image of ordinary encounters—a clinician and a patient talking through options, a family deciding whether to use a test, a community debating a new policy. The future of medicine will be forged in those conversations as much as in any lab. My deepest hope is that as biology becomes more programmable, our commitment to human dignity becomes more unwavering, not less.

Inspirational Quotes

The real revolution in medicine is not that we can change biology, but that we can choose to change it in service of compassion rather than power.

Epilogue:

Choosing Our Future, Cell by Cell

By the time you reach this page, you have traveled through many layers of the new medical era. You have visited the double helix of DNA and the bustling communities of the microbiome, watched immune cells retrained for battle, and seen organs reduced to chips and reconstructed in dishes. You have stepped into hospital rooms where gene therapies are infused, into homes where biotech arrives in small cardboard boxes, and into public debates about fairness, risk, and responsibility. The picture that emerges is not a single device or discovery, but a woven tapestry of tools and ideas that together are changing our relationship with our own biology.

It can be tempting, after such a tour, to feel either dizzy with optimism or weighed down by concern. On one side, there is the vision of a future where many diseases that haunt us today—certain cancers, genetic disorders, some forms of organ failure—are prevented, tamed, or cured. Where aging is gentler, where diagnosis is earlier and more precise, and where therapies are tailored rather than blunt. On the other side, there is the recognition that technology has never been evenly shared or perfectly managed. Biotech can just as easily deepen inequalities, invite new forms of surveillance, and narrow our ideas of what kinds of bodies and minds are welcome.

The truth, as always, lies in how we choose to use what we have built. Genes, cells, microbes, and algorithms do not carry moral direction on their own. They are tools—astonishingly powerful tools—that can be aimed in different ways. We can direct them toward compassion, fairness, and the relief of suffering, or we can allow them to drift toward profit, status, and control. The difference will not be decided in a single law or landmark trial; it will emerge from thousands of decisions made by researchers, clinicians, companies, policymakers, and ordinary people over many years.

You are part of that story whether or not you ever touch a pipette or write a line of code. You are part of it when you consider enrolling in a trial, when you read a headline about a new therapy and choose how to respond, when you vote for leaders who shape health policy, and when you listen to friends and family wrestling with diagnoses and options. You are part of it when you question whether access is fair, when you ask for clear explanations, and when you support efforts to bring effective care to those who are usually last in line. Biotech may be complex, but the values that should guide it—dignity, empathy, justice—are as old as human community.

If there is one thread that runs through this book, it is that medicine is no longer something that simply happens to us. More than ever before, it is something we shape, together. The same tools that allow us to edit genes or train immune cells also invite us to edit assumptions and train institutions—to reexamine who gets to decide, who is included in the conversation, and what goals we are pursuing. That work is slower and less glamorous than a breakthrough headline, but it is just as important.

The next fifty years of medicine will not arrive as a finished package. They will be built cell by cell, policy by policy, story by story. They will be written in the language of DNA and data, but also in the language of bedside conversations, community meetings, and quiet acts of care. As you close this book, my hope is not that you remember every technical detail, but that you carry forward a deeper sense of agency and responsibility. Biotechnology is giving us new power over life; our task is to ensure that we use that power in ways that honor life, rather than diminish it.

What we do next—individually and together—will decide whether "biotech breakthroughs" become a phrase that evokes only wonder, or one that also carries regret. The future is not yet fixed. It is, like a cell in the process of becoming, full of potential, waiting for instructions.

About the Author

Laura Lee is a writer, creative entrepreneur, and digital visionary whose work lives at the crossroads of feeling and possibility. Growing up in a quiet town where stories were a lifeline, she learned early how words can heal, connect, and open doors to new ways of seeing.

As the founder of a thriving digital design agency, Laura has guided brands and creators in shaping identities that are not only beautiful, but honest—rooted in clarity, purpose, and heart. Her writing carries the same signature: personal yet universal, grounded in themes of authenticity, healing, and intentional living.

For Laura, design is less about decoration and more about intention, and love is less about romance and more about telling the truth—first to ourselves, and then to the world. Through her books, online platforms, and creative consulting, she helps others reclaim their voice, honor their story, and build lives that align with their deepest values.

This book is a continuation of that work: a quiet companion for self-discovery and a gentle guide to remembering who you are, even in a world that constantly invites you to forget.

www.ingramcontent.com/pod-product-compliance
Lightning Source LLC
LaVergne TN
LVHW050303210926
848481LV00014BA/807